CAMBRIDGE LIBRARY COLLECTION

Books of enduring scholarly value

History of Medicine

It is sobering to realise that as recently as the year in which On the Origin of Species was published, learned opinion was that diseases such as typhus and cholera were spread by a 'miasma', and suggestions that doctors should wash their hands before examining patients were greeted with mockery by the profession. The Cambridge Library Collection reissues milestone publications in the history of Western medicine as well as studies of other medical traditions. Its coverage ranges from Galen on anatomical procedures to Florence Nightingale's common-sense advice to nurses, and includes early research into genetics and mental health, colonial reports on tropical diseases, documents on public health and military medicine, and publications on spa culture and medicinal plants.

Elizabeth Garrett Anderson

Elizabeth Garrett Anderson (1836–1917), physician, feminist and champion of women's medical education, played a key role in advancing the position of women in British professional life. Elizabeth's determination to qualify as a doctor, despite the many obstacles put in her way by the all-male medical establishment, was characteristic of her strong sense of purpose. Eventually joining the medical register in 1865, she established the St Mary's Dispensary for Women and Children in 1866, adding ten beds five years later as it became the New Hospital for Women. Staffed only by women, the hospital later moved to a purpose-built site on Euston Road and offered clinical experience to students at the London School of Medicine for Women. Through her tireless efforts, her chosen profession was opened to women. This 1939 biography by her daughter Louisa (1873–1943), herself a distinguished physician, is presented largely through Elizabeth's own letters.

Cambridge University Press has long been a pioneer in the reissuing of out-of-print titles from its own backlist, producing digital reprints of books that are still sought after by scholars and students but could not be reprinted economically using traditional technology. The Cambridge Library Collection extends this activity to a wider range of books which are still of importance to researchers and professionals, either for the source material they contain, or as landmarks in the history of their academic discipline.

Drawing from the world-renowned collections in the Cambridge University Library and other partner libraries, and guided by the advice of experts in each subject area, Cambridge University Press is using state-of-the-art scanning machines in its own Printing House to capture the content of each book selected for inclusion. The files are processed to give a consistently clear, crisp image, and the books finished to the high quality standard for which the Press is recognised around the world. The latest print-on-demand technology ensures that the books will remain available indefinitely, and that orders for single or multiple copies can quickly be supplied.

The Cambridge Library Collection brings back to life books of enduring scholarly value (including out-of-copyright works originally issued by other publishers) across a wide range of disciplines in the humanities and social sciences and in science and technology.

Elizabeth Garrett Anderson

1836–1917

Louisa Garrett Anderson

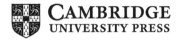

CAMBRIDGE
UNIVERSITY PRESS

University Printing House, Cambridge, CB2 8BS, United Kingdom

Cambridge University Press is part of the University of Cambridge.
It furthers the University's mission by disseminating knowledge in the pursuit of
education, learning and research at the highest international levels of excellence.

www.cambridge.org
Information on this title: www.cambridge.org/9781108079280

© in this compilation Cambridge University Press 2015

This edition first published 1939
This digitally printed version 2015

ISBN 978-1-108-07928-0 Paperback

ELIZABETH GARRETT ANDERSON

1836–1917

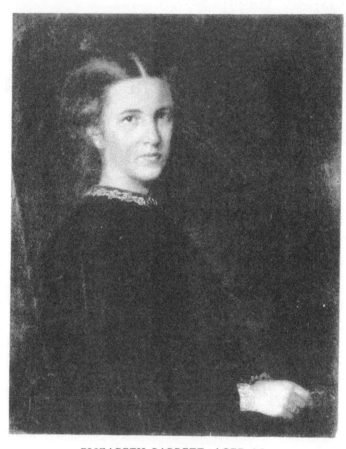

ELIZABETH GARRETT, AGED 30
from the portrait by Laura Herford, 1866

ELIZABETH
GARRETT ANDERSON

1836–1917

by her daughter

LOUISA
GARRETT ANDERSON

FABER AND FABER LIMITED
24 Russell Square
London

First published in April Mcmxxxix
by Faber and Faber Limited
24 Russell Square London W.C.1
Printed in Great Britain by
Latimer Trend & Co Ltd Plymouth
All Rights Reserved

This record of their grandmother
has been written for
Colin and Donald, Diana and Hermione
and for the
Heirs of her Spirit,
for those who follow where she led,
that they may know her better

PREFACE

Without the help of my brother, Alan, this *Life* would not have been written. He remembered what I forgot and improved what I wrote. He and Colin have made this 'our' book and I shall not thank them in print.

Letters written by Elizabeth Garrett to Miss Emily Davies were given to me by her niece, Miss Margaret Llewelyn Davies, and they provide the account of Elizabeth's struggle for medical training. Miss Llewelyn Davies also read the manuscript through, identifying many references in the letters. She could not have been more encouraging or kind.

To Lady Stephen I owe most generous help. Her accurate study of Miss Davies in *Emily Davies and Girton College* is a text-book of the early years of the women's movement, and by her permission it has been used constantly in the preparation of this book. Some of the letters to Miss Davies from Elizabeth Garrett and others written by Miss Davies have been printed already in Lady Stephen's book. Her suggestions, those of an ex-

Preface

perienced and successful biographer, have been extremely useful. By permission of Mrs. Oliver Strachey, extracts from Florence Nightingale's *Cassandra*, published in full in *The Cause*, 1928, have been included. Mr. William Hern, who was a medical student at the Middlesex Hospital in the eighteen-sixties, contributed information about the medical staff and the surgical technique at that time; and from Dr. H. Campbell Thomson's excellent account in *The Story of the Middlesex Hospital Medical School* more information of the same kind was obtained. Sir Edward Penton, K.B.E., searched the minutes of the East London Hospital for Children, Shadwell (renamed Princess Elizabeth of York Hospital for Children) for references to my parents who met in the hospital in 1869. Lady Stewart-Wilson, daughter of Professor Tulloch of St. Andrews, and Professor R. K. Hannay, Historiographer Royal of Scotland, have been most kind in collecting information about the University of St. Andrews in 1864.

Among the early friends of medical women, few were as courageous and sympathetic as Viscountess Amberley, and I am indebted to the Earl and Countess Russell and the Hogarth Press for permission to quote from *The Amberley Papers*. Thanks are due to the Editors of the *British Medical Journal*, the *Lancet*, *The Times*, and the *Spectator*, also to the Proprietors of *Punch* to quote from these papers.

At the London School of Medicine for Women and

the Elizabeth Garrett Anderson Hospital for Women no
trouble has been too great in helping to collect material.
Miss Elizabeth Bolton, C.B.E., M.D., Dean of the
School and Senior Surgeon at the Hospital, and Lady
Robertson, Chairman of the Hospital Committee, read
the chapters dealing with both institutions and made
helpful suggestions. Miss Burt, Librarian at the School,
supplied minute books and reports. To the relatives of
Dr. Sophia Jex-Blake I owe much. Miss Jex-Blake and
her sisters and Dr. Arthur Jex-Blake, F.R.C.P., read in
typescript the section dealing with their aunt and the
foundation by her of the London School of Medicine
for Women, and they gave permission for the inclusion
of an unpublished letter by Dr. Sophia Jex-Blake, whose
portrait by Samuel Lawrence has been reproduced by
kind permission of the Royal Society of Medicine. Sir
St. Clair Thomson has supplied vivid memories of his
master, Lord Lister, to whom more than fifty years
ago he acted as house-surgeon.

The list of acknowledgements, long as it is, would be
altogether incomplete without adding my appreciation
of the help received throughout from Miss F. C. Johnson, M.A. and Miss L. M. Brooks, O.B.E., who have spent
much time over the manuscript, and to Miss Mona
Wilson, who read the last chapter under circumstances
which made this service difficult to give.

The proofs have been corrected by Miss F. C. Johnson
and Dr. H. Campbell Thomson.

Preface

Two appendices have been added.

Appendix I includes press extracts, and four verses from Rudyard Kipling's poem, *The Song of the Women,* are reprinted by permission of Mrs. Rudyard Kipling and of Messrs. Methuen & Co.

Appendix II consists of short biographical notes on people mentioned in the text. Mrs. Douglas Carter (Alice Le Mesurier), professional researcher, whose investigations have been most helpful, is responsible for most of them. In many I have used her notes without alteration; the information was collected from the *Dictionary of National Biography*, by permission of the Oxford University Press, and from other sources which as far as possible have been indicated.

LOUISA GARRETT ANDERSON
  Penn, Bucks
  January 1939

CONTENTS

PREFACE   *page* 9
CH. I. THE POSITION OF WOMEN IN ENGLAND,
        1836   17
    II. THE GARRETT FAMILY   25
    III. EMILY DAVIES   39
    IV. MEDICAL TRAINING   50
    V. THE PARIS M.D.   120
    VI. INTERLUDES 1870: FRANCO-PRUSSIAN
         WAR; FIRST LONDON SCHOOL
         BOARD ELECTION   137
    VII. ENGAGEMENT   163
    VIII. EARLY YEARS OF MARRIAGE—THE
          NURSERY   188
    IX. THE LONDON SCHOOL OF MEDICINE
         FOR WOMEN   206
    X. THE NEW HOSPITAL FOR WOMEN   241
    XI. THE BRITISH MEDICAL ASSOCIATION   251
    XII. RETIREMENT   264

13

Contents

APP. I. MISCELLANEOUS   *page* 279

II. BIOGRAPHICAL NOTES   288

INDEX   315

ILLUSTRATIONS

ELIZABETH GARRETT, AGED 30   *frontispiece*
    from the portrait by Laura Herford, 1866

MR. AND MRS. NEWSON GARRETT WITH LOUIE
    AND ELIZABETH (ELIZABETH AGED 2) *facing page* 26
    from a painting by an unknown artist, 1838

SARAH EMILY DAVIES, AGED 37   42

J. G. S. ANDERSON AS A YOUNG MAN   134

ELIZABETH GARRETT ANDERSON, AGED 40   196

SOPHIA JEX-BLAKE, AGED 25   210
    from the portrait by Samuel Lawrence

ELIZABETH GARRETT ANDERSON, AGED 54   230

ELIZABETH GARRETT ANDERSON, AGED 73   270
    from a photograph by Olive Edis, F.R.P.S. (Mrs. E.
    H. Galsworthy)

15

THE POSITION OF WOMEN
IN ENGLAND, 1836

⋙⋗⋙●⋘⋖⋘

The women's movement in England took shape about the middle of the nineteenth century. Fifty years earlier, Mary Wollstonecraft horrified her contemporaries by writing *A Vindication of the Rights of Women*, 1792. Of all those who have worked for the women's movement, she stands apart, a genius and a prophet. She wrote as the champion of women, half the human species, 'labouring under a yoke which through the records of time' had degraded them. She appealed to women for worthy conceptions of self-respect and to men to break the chains from women and to accept from them rational fellowship instead of slavish obedience. 'It is time', she wrote, 'to strike a revolution in female manners: to restore their lost dignity and make them labour, and by reforming themselves reform the world.' If women took exercise, she said, their bodies would become strong and a reasonable education would cultivate their minds. Why should they not enter spheres of paid work, instead of eating out their hearts in idleness? 'Women might cer-

The Position of Women in England, 1836

tainly study the art of healing and be physicians as well as nurses,' and again, 'Women must have a civic existence in the State, married or single.' 'Let woman share the rights and she will emulate the virtues of man.' No wonder England was shocked. Mary Wollstonecraft was far in advance of her time and her programme is not completed yet.

Five years later she died, and for half a century the position of women changed little. Then, gradually, the humanitarian movement awakened dull consciences and the idea dawned in lesser minds than that of Mary Wollstonecraft that women had rights as well as men. The organized women's movement started about 1850 and was at first controlled by middle-class women who thought mainly of the needs of women in their own class. Later, when the parliamentary franchise was extended (1867), the demand for votes for women began and working-class women co-operated actively. Many other reforms took place during Elizabeth Garrett's life, but she gave untiring support and her whole strength to the women's movement. 'No one has time for everything,' she said, and, 'the passion of my life is to help women.'

It may be well to describe shortly the position of middle-class women in England in 1836, the year Elizabeth Garrett was born.

The much discussed case of Mrs. Caroline Norton occurred that year and directed public attention to the

The Position of Women in England, 1836

legal disabilities of married women. Mrs. Norton left her husband on account of his cruelty: she could not bring an action against him, employ counsel, keep possession of money she inherited or earned, nor force him to tell her where he had sent the children. The rights of a husband over the children of the marriage were absolute and at his death he could leave them under a guardianship which did not include their mother.

Petitions were organized to alter these laws and the agitation started which finally secured the Equal Guardianship of Infants Act, 1839, and the Married Women's Property Act, 1870.

Although marriage had these disadvantages, most women wished to marry. As Florence Nightingale wrote, 'Marriage is the only chance (and it is but a chance) offered to women to escape from this death [idleness] and how eagerly and how ignorantly it is embraced.'

To remain single was thought a disgrace and at thirty an unmarried woman was called an old maid. Those who did not marry formed the problem of the superfluous woman. After their parents died, what could they do, where could they go? If they had a brother, as unwanted and permanent guests, they might live in his house. Some had to maintain themselves and then, indeed, difficulty arose. A hundred years ago the only paid occupation open to a gentlewoman was to become a governess under despised conditions and at a miserable salary.

The Position of Women in England, 1836

None of the professions were open to women; there were no women in Government offices; secretarial work was not done by them. Even nursing was disorganized and disreputable until Florence Nightingale recreated it as a profession by founding the Nightingale School of Nursing in 1860.

Men were believed to dislike 'blue-stockings', so that parents thought the serious education of their daughters superfluous: deportment, music and a little French would see them through. 'To learn arithmetic will not help my daughter to find a husband,' was a common maternal point of view; 'Be good, sweet maid, and let who will be clever,' the prevalent adage. A governess at home, for a short period, was the usual fate of the girls. Their brothers might go to public schools and the university, but 'home' was considered the right place for their sisters. Some parents sent their daughters to a finishing-school, but good schools for girls did not exist. Their teachers were untrained and ill-educated. No public examinations accepted female candidates. Schoolgirls did not play games. It would be disastrous to let their faces tan with the sun and it was undesirable that they should grow strong and muscular. When weather permitted they walked in pairs in a 'crocodile', sunshades, veils and 'clouds' being in constant use. High buttoned boots were worn, and gloves even in the garden. Their hair and their clothes prevented active exercise. Voluminous petticoats and constricting bands hampered them; as they grew up, their skirts touched the ground. Crinolines gave way to bustles, but the number of petticoats and the length of skirts remained unaltered. 'Woollen next the skin' was the rule, and stays became bonier and bonier as age increased. A waist of 21 inches was desired; no measurement over 25 inches was permitted. To look languid and anaemic was thought correct for a girl. It gave her a refined appearance. No doubt their dull lives and uncomfortable clothes were responsible for some of the fashionable complaints from which women of the period suffered—depression, the vapours, hysteria and fainting fits. Whether well or ailing, daughters at home were expected to be 'bright and gay', ready at any time to drive with mamma or to amuse papa. Their lives were of no account. In the morning they turned over photograph albums or did needlework, sitting together in the parlour. If a woman had gifts she must not use them: if she had knowledge, she must hide it.

Writers of the period preach the inferiority of women and their need for self-repression, patience and resignation. Above all they must avoid any sign of superior information, men disliking this so much. The writings of Mrs. Ellis had a great vogue. 'It is the privilege of a married woman', she wrote, 'to be able to show by the most delicate attentions how much she feels her husband's superiority to herself not by mere personal services but by a respectful deference to his opinion, a

The Position of Women in England, 1836

willingly imposed silence when he speaks.' And again, 'Even a highly gifted woman must not exhibit the least disposition to presume upon such gifts for fear of raising her husband's jealousy of her importance.' A daughter at home had neither a latch-key nor money. She could go nowhere alone, a chaperon being indispensable.

Apart from want of education, inability to earn a reasonable salary, and legal injustice, there was the mental stigma. The moral, intellectual and physical inferiority of women to men was accepted almost universally. No one has expressed her resentment of this attitude with greater force than Florence Nightingale. Her home was cultured and wealthy; her education had been excellent; legal disabilities did not touch her; but since she was a 'young lady' she had to live in idleness, and at the age of thirty she longed to die. In 1852 she wrote a fragment, *Cassandra*, from which the following extracts are taken: 'To have no food for our heads, no food for our hearts, no food for our activity, is that nothing? If we have no food for the body how do we cry out ... how all the newspapers talk of it ...! Death from Starvation! But suppose we were to put a paragraph in *The Times*— Death of Thought from Starvation ... how people would stare...! We have nothing to do which raises us ... We can never pursue any object for a single two hours.' 'Jesus Christ raised women above the condition of mere slaves, mere ministers to the passions of the man, raised them by his sympathy, to be ministers of God. He gave

22

them moral activity. But the Age, the World, Humanity, must give them the means to exercise this moral activity, must give them intellectual cultivation, spheres of action.' 'There is perhaps no century where the woman shows so meanly as in this.'

Summed up, then, the position of English middle-class women during the first half of the nineteenth century was very restricted and exceedingly dull. They were not trained to do anything and they had no responsibilities. They possessed none of the rights of citizenship beyond that of paying rates and taxes. They could not vote at municipal or parliamentary elections. This state of affairs excited little comment. It was accepted by men and women alike. It was not thought to be cruel or unjust; it was taken for granted until the case of Caroline Norton occurred, followed some years later by the protesting voices of Barbara Leigh Smith (later Mme Bodichon), Emily Davies, Elizabeth Garrett and others. Gradually supporters appeared and the movement took shape.

Perhaps increased ease of travel helped. In 1836 almost every one remained where his work took him and mixed with a small unchanging group of people with ideas to match. In the eighteen-thirties railways were beginning and fast coaches were near the end of their short life, but all except the wealthy stayed at home or suffered on their journeys what we should call extreme discomfort and delay. The misery of travel except by the best coaches on the best roads must have been great. Jolting over ruts a foot or more deep, luggage might be lost and outside passengers might die from exposure. With the railways travel became easy and ideas began to stir. Decades later the advent of the tricycle (1880) and the bicycle (1890) undoubtedly helped the emancipation of women. They made dress reform necessary. The coat and skirt and small sailor hat appeared. On their bicycles girls escaped from their chaperon and left their fainting fits and vapours behind.

2

THE GARRETT FAMILY

>>>◗◖<<

In 1836, when Elizabeth Garrett was born, the world
did not treat her sex kindly, but to a child the home is
all important and in hers love and justice reigned, boys
and girls sharing everything equally.

Elizabeth's parents, Mr. and Mrs. Newson Garrett,
were Suffolk people. For generations his forbears had
been gunsmiths and makers of agricultural implements
in different parts of the county. In 1675 a Richard
Garrett carried on the trade of edge-tool-maker at
Ufford, Suffolk, and somewhat later at Glemham a
Garrett worked as blade-smith. In 1778 another Richard
Garrett (grandfather of Newson), coming to Leiston,
married the daughter and inherited the business of Mr.
Newson, agricultural tool-maker in that place. In 1807
Newson Garrett's elder brother Richard, sixth in the
direct series of name and trade, was born. During his
life the Leiston works prospered as Richard Garrett &
Sons, and before his death, 1866, they did a large export
trade.

The Garrett Family

Newson Garrett was born in 1812. He and Richard married sisters, Louisa and Elizabeth Dunnell. During the early years of their marriage, Newson and Louisa lived in London, with or near her parents. During this period three children were born—Louisa Maria (Louie), February 1835; on 9 June 1836 Elizabeth, and in 1837 a son who died in infancy.

The 'Happy Family' group reproduced opposite is said to be a good portrait of the Garretts in 1838. This ambitious painting was commissioned by Newson Garrett when he was twenty-six and far from rich. It shows that he meant to found a family and that he had courage.

One of Elizabeth's earliest recollections was the state visit of Queen Victoria and Prince Albert to the opera after their marriage in 1840. Mr. Garrett insisted that Elizabeth should see the procession. 'Dear Mother' expostulated, the hour was late and the child asleep. Her father had vision: 'Nonsense,' he said, 'the child *must* see it. She will remember it all her life.' On his shoulder Elizabeth was taken to the window and saw the crowds and the lights, and she passed the picture on to her children.

Soon afterwards the Garretts went to live at Aldeburgh on the coast of Suffolk. The journey was by sea, the usual route at that date, and great was the discomfort of landing young children and furniture from open boats. In Tudor times Aldeburgh had been an important

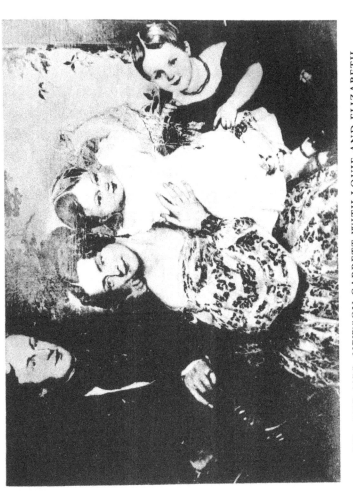

MR. AND MRS. NEWSON GARRETT WITH LOUIE AND ELIZABETH
(ELIZABETH AGED 2 YEARS)

from a painting by an unknown artist, 1838

place; it had contributed five ships to fight the Spanish Armada, and in another crisis a Martello tower had been built to resist Napoleon. Also it was the birthplace of the poet George Crabbe. These were its contributions to history. In 1840 it was a sleepy place; fishing was the industry and there was little society and few visitors. All that the sea had left between the marshes and the shingle was the Moot Hall and a main and a back street stretching half a mile parallel to the sea.

The Garretts settled in a roomy house at the top of Church Hill. It is not known how Mr. Garrett financed his start as householder and business man. Mrs. Garrett had some money and perhaps Newson's father gave him a share in the family estate. Anyhow what he lacked in cash he made up for in character and ability. Although the Aldeburgh of 1840 was a queer place for an ambitious man to choose for founding a business and a family, he made his way and throve. Every two years a new baby joined the circle until finally there were six daughters and four sons. No wonder Mrs. Garrett's hands were full. The nursery overflowed. She washed, dressed and fed the last baby, scrutinized her whole establishment and kept a minute account of expenditure. One of her petty cash books has survived with entries from day to day: Teddy's boots 4/-: Elizabeth, sundries at school 13/6: Alice's tooth 1/-: toll gates 7d, dd. 6d, dd. 3d: milk for calf 1/5: donkies 3/6: 700 snails [for slaughter, 2d. a hundred] 1/2 Edmund and Alice. It is comforting to read amongst these items 3/- pr. of chickens, 3/6 pr. of ducks, etc., although to feed ten children even with chickens at 3/- a pair must have been an effort. The dairy and pastry-making were in her hands and she overlooked the laundry. Her husband needed her help. She advised him and calmed those with whom he quarrelled. He was warm-hearted but impetuous and the bracing air made people quarrelsome. Disputes with the vicar, Mr. Dowler, became a byword. Sometimes, for weeks on end, Mr. Garrett took his family to chapel: then the trouble was patched up and they returned to church. At Christmas-time a distribution of poultry took place. 'Why, Mother dear, surely you know that I quarrelled with that fellow?' said Newson, as he saw the offending name pinned to the breast of a turkey. 'Patience me, yes, of course I do, Father dear, but that doesn't make any difference.' Indeed the village began to think that a little quarrel with Mr. Garrett in the autumn might increase the size of the gift at Christmas. Mrs. Garrett's handwriting was neat and clear. Important words were underlined. She made no mistakes in spelling or grammar. It is not surprising that 'dear Mother' often received a summons to the business room where she wrote and sometimes composed letters for her husband. Those which have survived are excellent, but it must be admitted that her letters to her family were dull. On principle she avoided news as allied to gossip, and scriptural allusions and texts predominated with comments on the weather or the health of those at home. She had an excellent constitution, was a good business woman and very religious in the evangelical school. She took in Spurgeon's *Sermons* and was a strict Sabbatarian. A critic of the clergyman and a constant member of his congregation, she was the pillar of the church in Aldeburgh.

Mr. Garrett respected his wife greatly and was proud of her piety. In later life, when he went abroad, he would attend divine service every Sunday although he could not understand a word, in order that he might tell 'dear Mother' that he had 'been to church'.

It is doubtful whether she owned a cheque book until, in old age, she became a widow. Then a new pleasure dawned as she wrote cheques for her grandchildren, for her daughter's hospital or for the conversion of the Jews.

Mr. Garrett lived before the age of general education. It is not known that he went to school, and perhaps his respect for education was the greater from the thought of what he had missed. His spelling was phonetic and his handwriting illegible. Spelling is not a sign of education. Newson could not spell, but he devised a cloak for this little defect. He wrote with a quill pen and when in doubt for a letter or two, the quill would dart forward in a thick continuous stroke until it reached letters on which he could rely. It was an excellent device but sometimes obscured his meaning. He became the active man for all business in Aldeburgh and the surrounding district. He founded and conducted maltings up the River

The Garrett Family

Alde at Snape, he owned a fleet of sailing barges, he founded gas works, he was partner in a brewery, he conducted a brickyard and built rows of houses of which he was the architect—Brudenell Terrace in ornamental brick being his masterpiece. He acted as agent for Lloyd's, he served as Justice of the Peace, and out of all this business in a remote and sleepy corner of England, he contrived to live well, to bring up and educate his family on a liberal scale and at his death to leave a modest fortune.

To return to earlier days, it became clear that Mrs. Garrett had too much to do. By the time Elizabeth was ten help with the elder girls was needed. Miss Edgeworth, a distant relative of Maria Edgeworth the novelist, commended herself to Mr. and especially to Mrs. Garrett by her poverty, friendlessness and piety. She was engaged as resident governess. During a life of dependence, poor soul, no doubt she had needed protective colouring. Her opinions like her religion quickly matched those of Mrs. Garrett. Sometimes Mr. Garrett grew impatient. 'Bless my soul, Miss Edgeworth, you said just the opposite a moment ago.' Miss Edgeworth was shameless. 'I had not heard dear Mrs. Garrett's opinion when I spoke last.'

Miss Edgeworth received £25 a year. She had her meals with the family. She never took a holiday. She shared a bedroom with the elder girls and crept fully dressed behind the curtains of the four-poster at night, to emerge next morning in the same genteel condition.

She was untrained and uneducated. She possessed neither imagination nor humour, nor the physique to grapple with healthy and intelligent children in the schoolroom or out of it. She relied on three books:

(1) Mangnall's *Questions* (*Historical and Miscellaneous*).

(2) Slater's *Sententiae Chronologicae*, in which consonants stood for figures and appropriate sentences helped students to remember dates.

(3) Tables of Irregular French Verbs.

In the afternoon Miss Edgeworth and her charges walked for an hour. Two roads led from Aldeburgh, one to Leiston, the other to Saxmundham. They were taken in turn: one mile out and then back. The children might not run, play, pick flowers nor even talk to one another. Miss Edgeworth listened to the recitation of irregular French verbs or to answers of questions from Mangnall's compendium of learning. From this work, an extract may explain the views of the pupils upon their governess and her text-book:

History of England. Richard III. 'He waded to the throne through the blood of his nearest relations . . . but as king he managed the helm with success.' To us this suggests *1066 and All That*; but they were too close to think it funny.

The children soon found to their delight that they could cause Miss Edgeworth discomfort by asking questions the answers to which she had not prepared. By the time Louie was fifteen and Elizabeth thirteen, they were out of hand and they were sent to school.

Mr. Garrett did not spare trouble or expense over the education of his children. He insisted that they should have the best he could obtain, boys and girls alike. The eldest son had a tutor at home and went into the army. Edmund was sent to the City of London School and Sam to Rugby and Cambridge where he became a Fellow of Peterhouse, in later life being a leading solicitor in London and President of the Law Society.

To his daughters, Mr. Garrett opened the windows of the world by sending them to boarding-school and, later, helping them to continue the friendships of their school-days. He took trouble in the choice of their school. Finally it was decided that Louie and Elizabeth should go to an 'Academy for the Daughters of Gentlemen' at Blackheath, kept by Miss Browning and her sister, aunts of the poet. Their father drove the girls in the dogcart to join the coach on the main road, four miles from Alde-burgh. Then, hoisted to the box-seat, beside the driver, sixpence extra, they bowled away to Ipswich to take the train to London.

Mr. Garrett stipulated that his daughters should have all extras at the school, including a hot bath once a week. Such cleanliness made them marked girls. They were called 'the bathing Garretts'. Every Saturday night the laundry tub was placed before the kitchen fire and, screened by a towel-horse, they sat in it by turn. In

ˈfairness to the school it must be remembered that in
1849 even in large houses bathrooms were unusual and
the installation of one at Windsor Castle two years earlier
was due to the reforming zeal of Prince Albert.

In another department of hygiene Miss Browning was
in advance of her time She believed in fresh air and
often the door of a stuffy classroom would open. Miss
Browning was large and her figure filled the doorway
making a gay patch of colour, as she liked to wear
ribbons of bright and varied hues. 'De l'air, de l'air,'
she cried and a governess hastened to open a window.
French had to be spoken always. It was the rule of the
school and Elizabeth gained a fluent knowledge of the
language as spoken in Blackheath. Miss Browning and
her sister often mentioned 'our nephew Robert' and
gave their pupils the impression that he might call at
any time, but he never came. The teaching may have
been poor, indeed 'the stupidity of the teachers' was
remembered by Elizabeth 'with shudders', but the girls
left school thirsty for knowledge and with friends who
influenced their lives—not a bad record for any school.
Perhaps Miss Edgeworth may be allowed to share the
credit—at any rate Mangnall's *Questions* and Blackheath
made the girls eager to use their brains. After two years
at Blackheath Louie and Elizabeth left, their education
considered at an end. Soon after leaving school they
visited the Great Exhibition which Prince Albert organized in Hyde Park in 1851. Uncle Richard, owner of the

The Garrett Family

Leiston works, gave them tips and we can picture them, keen sightseers, full skirts billowing over crinolines, poke bonnets with lace behind and roses under the brims, shawls draped on their shoulders and each with a dainty parasol in one mittened hand while the other clasped the money. To the end of her life, as she strolled across Hyde Park, Elizabeth would say: 'the exhibition buildings came as far as this' or 'the glass covered that elm.'

Family life at Alde House was happy. Harmony reigned and the girls were devoted to one another, calling themselves 'the sisterhood'. Louie supplied spiritual grace, Elizabeth determination, Alice literary taste, Millicent and Josephine wit, and Agnes, who did not marry, motherliness. All possessed public spirit and an intense desire to help other women. The girls had much simple gaiety in which cousins joined. In the winter they went to dances, often travelling in a farm cart with straw on the floor.

From 1850 to 1870 Newson Garrett was at his prime and usually his affairs prospered, but as happens with sanguine, progressive people, his growing business from time to time needed more help than his banker was inclined to supply. Then indeed his optimism turned to gloom; expenses were cut down; the children learned the nutritive value of Suffolk dumpling without its familiar beef. Millicent was recalled from school; the removal of the family to a smaller house was considered. But the crisis passed, beef reappeared and Milly went back to school. In 1852, at the age of forty, Mr. Garrett was the leading man in Aldeburgh and at this time he built Alde House, a substantial mansion surrounded by gardens and paddocks. It had stables, granaries, a dairy, glass-houses, piggeries, a large kitchen-garden, an ice-house, a laundry, and a Turkish Bath which the coachman called 'Master's Sweatin' House'. If old servants are the hall-mark of a good master, Mr. Garrett was pure gold. Lambert, the coachman, Alderton, the gardener, and Barham who 'did for the pigs' had been in his service for a generation when his grandchildren dawned upon them. Lambert was impressive, a tall man with a large nose, he wore a red waistcoat with sleeves, a green coat turning yellow and tarnished brass buttons. When Lambert was on the box of the brougham, which had a fusty smell, he wore a pointed tall hat like a stage highwayman's. His dictatorial manner kept children at a distance. Newson used to open the French window of the dining-room and bellow. Soon Lambert would appear with Polly, a fidgety mare of some breeding but aged as her rider then was. Newson climbed on to the mounting-block. 'Why don't you hold the mare still while I get on, Lambert?' 'Why don't you get on while I holds the mare still?'

Naturally a man of Newson's character attracted anecdotes, in youth and age. In a black north-easter, when the beachmen said they could not launch the lifeboat, he put them on their mettle by climbing into the boat with one of the children in his arms. The boat was launched without these passengers. To sailing ships Aldeburgh Bay was dangerous, and in the winter of 1855 seventeen wrecks occurred with much loss of life. Mr. Garrett received the official thanks of the Royal National Lifeboat Institution for his services.

At Alde House Newson said grace before lunch and dinner. He had two graces, one long—the familiar one—and the other short—a blow on the table with the carving-knife and 'Thank God—Amen'.

Before breakfast Mrs. Garrett read prayers and a chapter from the Bible; this was unusual, as to read prayers was a male prerogative, but it had happened long ago that Newson almost at the end of reading one long chapter had turned two pages at once and fallen into the beginning of another, so he closed his reading with the grace slightly modified, 'For what we have already received may the Lord make us thankful,' and was never allowed to read prayers again. It seemed to me hard, but it interested me even as a child to learn that in her own department my grandmother ruled without appeal or complaint. And so, with spectacles adjusted and the great Bible before her and in a voice suited to the occasion, Mrs. Garrett conducted family prayers.

In 1857, at the age of twenty-two, Louie married James Smith, the brother of school friends. Henceforth she lived in London and offered constant hospitality to her family. Elizabeth, aged twenty-one, took her place at home as eldest daughter. In the mornings she worked at Latin and arithmetic, sometimes under the guidance of a tutor who was coaching her brother for the army. She helped the younger children with their lessons, being 'almost maternal' in her attitude to them, as Millicent noted later. On Sunday evenings she collected her brothers and sisters and talked to them of 'things in general', principally of world affairs. Elizabeth sat on the drawing-room sofa, little George, the youngest, might sleep on her knee, the others listened attentively. She spoke to them about the Hungry Forties, the Potato Famine in Ireland, and the Crimean War. Had not their father burst into the dining-room, waving *The Times*, as he exclaimed, 'Heads up and shoulders down! Sebastopol is taken!'? She told them of the Indian Mutiny and spoke of Italy saved from the grasp of Austria by Garibaldi, whom she admired greatly.

Mr. Newson Garrett took a keen interest in politics and labelled himself a Conservative until, in the early sixties, he became a Liberal to the consternation of the Conservative member, Sir Fitzroy Kelly. Newson's change in party allegiance increased a coolness that existed between himself and his brother Richard, who called him a Radical, and from this time forward they seldom met. Among the family political opinion was divided. Edmund was born and died a Conservative. Reform or change of any sort was anathema to him. To bear it at all needed his strong family affection but

37

fortunately his heart was warm. Millicent was an ardent Liberal and all the children, except Edmund, welcomed reform.

By 1859 Elizabeth had been at home eight years since her school days. The third daughter, Alice, was well able to take her place and the other girls were growing up. Elizabeth wanted to make room for them, and for herself she felt a growing need for wider interests and something worthy to do. With these thoughts in her mind, she left home on the visit which decided her future.

3

EMILY DAVIES

I t is usual nowadays to provide girls with pocket money;
in Elizabeth's youth their dress bills were paid but they
had no petty cash. Mr. Garrett held other views and
wishing his daughters to see the world, he gladly provided money for the purpose. Before Louie married, she
and Elizabeth had been to Gateshead twice to visit Jane
and Annie Crowe, school friends from Blackheath, and
through them had made acquaintance with Jane's friend
Emily Davies, daughter of the rector of Gateshead. In
1859, the Crowes asked Elizabeth to stay with them
again. She accepted with pleasure but she had no reason
to think anything decisive would result. Yet the influence
of Emily Davies proved to be to Elizabeth what conversion has been to others. Emily turned her vague aspirations into a precise plan and for ten years inspired and
led her.

In ambition for other women Emily Davies from
youth onwards was an intrepid reformer, in other matters very conservative. She objected to the whole posi-

39

tion of women. She realized that their education was miserable; they were helpless in the labour market; unjustly treated by the law; their mental attitude was suited to a harem; they were slaves and clung to their fetters. To claim that at this stage she, the unassuming daughter of the rector of Gateshead, determined to alter these conditions, may be going too far. Yet, as she watched the world of women from the parlour of the rectory, her plans took shape. She resented her own lack of education and pondering over the lives of other women, found them empty and aimless. Speaking of them, she said, 'It was indeed no wonder that people who had not learnt to do anything, could not find anything to do.' No special trouble had been taken with her education although care had been lavished on her brothers. Her reading had been desultory and self-directed. She had had a governess at home. Later she had gained some practical experience in her father's parish. She was a convinced churchwoman and taught in the Sunday-school and edited the parish magazine, devoting much care to it. Her father made her write essays for him—perhaps the best bit of education she had. At any rate she determined to write good English prose and demanded from herself clear expression, few adjectives, no split infinitives or superfluous words. Throughout life she was an opportunist, feeling her way step by step. She had uncanny foresight and great determination. Gradually ideas shaped themselves. Better education must be provided for women and she decided that the professions, especially medicine, ought to be open to them. She did not herself feel suited to be a pioneer in medicine; for this part of her programme she needed a lieutenant. She meant to obtain good schools for girls with educated and qualified teachers. Examining bodies must accept women for public examinations and university education become accessible to them. Her father and brothers were scholars but scholarship for women was not her aim. She wanted university training and professional experience as levers to raise the whole position of women.

These views were most unusual in the orthodox circle to which she belonged, and she found no one in whom she could confide until in 1858 she went with a brother, who was ill and soon to die, to Algiers. There she met two outstanding women, Mme Bodichon and her sister, Miss Annie Leigh Smith. Before her marriage Mme Bodichon, then Barbara Leigh Smith, had written with legal help a pamphlet summarizing the most important laws concerning women; and no doubt the success of this effort encouraged her. The three young women became friends and Emily's plans took more definite form. The Leigh Smiths belonged to a Unitarian family and it was part of their tradition that women should be well educated and free to use their powers in public service. The visit to Algiers was of recent occurrence when in 1859 Elizabeth Garrett came again to Gateshead.

Emily Davies

Miss Davies' appearance in early life was most misleading. She did not suggest personality or power. She seemed to be a rather plain, rather dim little person with mouse-coloured hair and conventional manners. She was not even ugly. Never was there a more complete disguise than Providence provided for Emily Davies until in old age character and ability printed themselves on her face.

In London, on her way to Gateshead, Elizabeth Garrett met Dr. Elizabeth Blackwell, an Englishwoman with an American qualification who had been placed on the first Medical Register automatically as she was practising in England when the Medical Act was passed in 1858. A slighting reference had been made to Dr. Blackwell at Alde House, and Elizabeth in defence suggested that her father should find out about Dr. Blackwell from his partner in business, Mr. Valentine Smith, who knew her through his cousin, Mme Bodichon. He did so, but there was a misunderstanding. Mr. Smith thought Elizabeth wanted an introduction to the lady and, at Mme Bodichon's house in London, they met. 'She assumed that I had made up my mind to follow her,' Elizabeth wrote later, 'I remember feeling very much confounded and as if I had been suddenly thrust into work that was too big for me.' In fact she was booked as a recruit. Also, she attended three lectures on 'Medicine as a Profession for Ladies' given by Dr. Blackwell in the Portman Rooms, Baker Street. The lecturer noted that 'the most

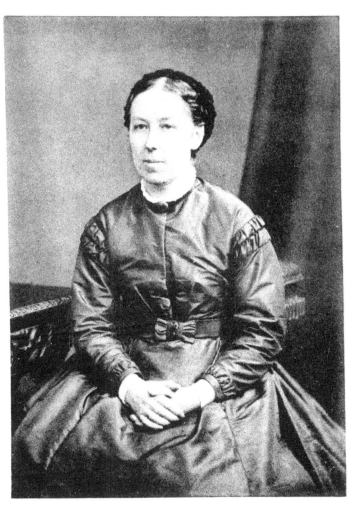

SARAH EMILY DAVIES, AGED 37

important listener was the bright, intelligent young lady whose interest in the study of medicine was then aroused —Miss Elizabeth Garrett.'

Elizabeth reached Gateshead undecided and yet tempted by the idea of medicine as a career. She was twenty-three years old, of medium height, her health was magnificent and she radiated vitality and energy. She rarely laughed and never was noisy. Her voice was pleasant and her manners unaffected and friendly. She was not eccentric. Miss Laura Herford's portrait, painted a few years later, shows a face that is grave and serene, a mouth determined if not stern, a clear complexion and auburn hair carried back from a broad forehead. Probably Miss Davies ran over these points in her unemotional way and decided that Elizabeth was the ideal pioneer.

They talked and talked, or possibly Miss Davies talked and Elizabeth listened and questioned. When Elizabeth came home she told her sister Alice, later Mrs. Herbert Cowell, as she climbed into the pony trap, that she was 'going to be a doctor'. To tell her parents was more difficult.

Frequent letters passed between Elizabeth and Miss Davies. Every move was reported to Gateshead; advice was asked constantly and sometimes taken. At what stage should she speak to her parents? She told her father first and on the whole the interview was satisfactory. He was surprised and puzzled, but Elizabeth felt sure he would support her eventually and that if she succeeded warm approval would follow. 'Success is all important,' she wrote:

E.G. to E.D.   *1860. Sunday afternoon*

'I have just concluded a satisfactory talk with Father on the medical subject. He was not at all disposed to oppose me actively and I shall be able to do as I think best in all essentials. He does not *like* it, I think, or at least, he would prefer my settling down into a douce young lady with no awkward energies, but when this is admitted to be impossible he will soon be reconciled to the other line, *if I succeed.* This is an all important point, of course, and it will nerve one up to almost any exertion to remember how far the cause is identified in the minds of one's own family with personal success: it ought not to be quite as much so as it is, considering the variety that there is among women and that though I may fail, it may be possible and most desirable for many others. I am very glad you do not tire of this subject, I like writing to you about it very much.'

With professional examinations in view Elizabeth redoubled her efforts to fill in the gaps of her education. Mr. Tate, the school master at Aldeburgh, coached her in Greek and Latin. She made him promise 'not to tell' in case her plans should fail. Miss Davies offered to criticize essays and papers sent by Elizabeth. This was welcomed and sermons, even Mr. Dowler's, provided material.

Emily Davies

E.G. to E.D.   *Ufford, 12 June 1860*
'Mr. Dowler's sermon last Sunday morning was so vile that I was moved to write some comments on it, by way of exercise in English. If you would look them over and correct them, at your leisure, I should be much obliged.

'If you can spare the time to send me a line by return, I should like to know if you would advise my not speaking to my father about my plans till you have heard of a doctor [to whom she could be apprenticed]. I think they may feel hurt, and in consequence rather angry, if when I do speak, they find my arrangements have been advanced as far as I could without consulting them. On the other hand the difficulty will be lessened by my being able to say that I know of a doctor who will take me as his pupil.'

Against some of the sentences Miss Davies wrote 'obscure', against others 'ungrammatical', while some were 'obscure and inelegant'. Evidently there was room for improvement and for years, in the matter of literary composition, this tuition by correspondence continued. No doubt the practice of sending papers to Miss Davies 'to cut up' and 'to criticize' was useful. To the Elizabeth of this period Emily Davies was a 'spiritual mother'.

E.G. to E.D.   *Aldeburgh, 15 June 1860*
'You would think my father awfully impetuous if you

knew him, and I can see how much it goes against him and how inconvenient it is.

'I have opened my letter to tell you of a long conversation that I have just had with my father. At first he was very discouraging, to my astonishment then, but now I fancy he did it as a forlorn hope to check me; he said the whole idea was so *disgusting* that he could not entertain it for a moment. I asked what there was to make doctoring more disgusting than nursing, which women were always doing, and which ladies had done publicly in the Crimea. He could not tell me. When I felt rather overcome with his opposition, I said as firmly as I could, that I must have this or something else, that I could not live without some real work, and then he objected that it would take seven years before I could practise. I said if it were seven years I should then be little more than 31 years old and able to work for twenty years probably. I think he will probably come round in time, I mean to renew the subject pretty often.'

E.G. to E.D.   *Aldeburgh, 26 June 1860*
'Thanks for the letters received this morning. I have had two hours talk with my mother about them and the result is, on the whole, sufficiently encouraging. They naturally feel very anxious about allowing me to enter upon such an untried life, and they are greatly puzzled as to the motive which can influence me. I cannot make them understand how impossible it would be for me to

live at home in happy idleness all my life. I believe they feel very nervous about either refusing or sanctioning it, but as long as I am very decided there is a good hope of their coming round.'

Mrs. Garrett did not accept new ideas readily. She was horrified at Elizabeth's suggestion and for some time her opposition increased. Thinking it a 'disgrace' that her daughter should leave home, she shut herself into her bedroom and made herself ill by crying. Elizabeth was much attached to her mother but clear-sighted about her limitations. Also she could distinguish imaginary illness from real, and imaginary grief from genuine. Mrs. Garrett's attitude distressed her but she did not take it seriously. She was staying with Louie in London when Mr. Garrett wrote, 'you will kill your mother if you go on,' and relatives advised her to give up her plans and to return home. Eventually a grudging assent was obtained.

Constant letters passed between Elizabeth and Miss Davies. All dealt with aspects of the subject which engrossed their minds—the cause, the position of women, examinations, and particularly every move Elizabeth made to forward her plans. It is doubtful whether success would ever have come without the guidance and advice given by Miss Davies, who, apart from this stream of letters, paid many visits to Alde House. Nobody has every quality, and a key to the heart of youth was not included among Miss Davies' great gifts when she was young. As founder and first mistress of Girton she was to win opportunity and hope for young women of all time, but faced by one or two ordinary girls she was shy and awkward. In old age she lost her shyness; with her complexion of alabaster, silver hair and the white Kashmir shawl over her shoulders she had presence and poise. The assurance of success made her gentle and accessible, and with some girls, notably her grand-nieces, she established the happiest friendship. When Miss Davies began to visit Alde House in 1860, time and success had not yet mellowed her, and it must be confessed that the younger Garretts were critical. Her manner was dry, snubbing, they thought, and Elizabeth's absorption in her became tiresome. The constant talk about education, examinations, medicine and women grew monotonous. After all, there were such things as picnics and parties, although apparently Miss Davies had not heard of them and Elizabeth was in danger of forgetting them. Indeed the cause absorbed them both, they wanted neither picnics nor parties.

Here is a picture of them during a visit to Alde House. Before the bedroom fire, the girls were brushing their hair. Emily was twenty-nine, Elizabeth twenty-three and Millicent thirteen. As they brushed, they debated. 'Women can get nowhere', said Emily, 'unless they are as well educated as men. I shall open the universities to them.' 'Yes,' agreed Elizabeth. 'We need education but we need an income too and we can't earn that without training and a profession. I shall start women in medicine. But what shall we do with Milly?' They agreed that she should get the parliamentary vote for women.

4

MEDICAL TRAINING

>>⊃●⊂<<

Newson Garrett knew no more than his daughter about medical training and they had no introductions to help their assault on a conservative profession. He did not like her scheme particularly and friends advised against it. Mrs. Garrett liked it even less and her opinion carried great weight with him. However, he could not let Elizabeth fight the first round without an ally, so in June 1860 he came to London and with his twenty-four-year-old daughter walked down Harley Street, calling on the leading medical consultants. The result was discouraging. 'Why not be a nurse?' said one of the doctors. 'Because I prefer to earn a thousand, rather than twenty pounds a year.' No one offered help or believed in her high aspiration. Some laughed, some were rude; but one good result followed. Opposition put Mr. Garrett on his mettle and, gradually, whatever he might say in private against Elizabeth's plans—perhaps to be primed with arguments in support of them—in public his daughter's cause became his own. No sacrifice of time or money deterred him. He made up his mind that THEY must succeed.

Miss Davies suggested that she and Elizabeth should call on Mrs. Russell Gurney, wife of the Recorder of London, who had promised Dr. Elizabeth Blackwell, then in America, to see any women who volunteered for medical training. An introduction was arranged through the Rev. Llewelyn Davies, and Mrs. Gurney delighted Elizabeth with her originality and charm.

E.G. to E.D.   *Aldeburgh, 28 June 1860*

'I shall come to London to hear if you have any plans for me. I should be very glad if you would go with me to see Mrs. Gurney. My father introduced the subject of women physicians yesterday at dinner, and he asked Sarah's [Mrs. Freeman, a cousin] opinion. She was quite against it, but not in an intelligent way, and my father felt this, I think, for he said that he must say he should prefer a woman attending his wife and daughters, if he could be thoroughly satisfied that she was qualified.'

As yet Elizabeth and her friends had not full confidence in Mr. Garrett as an ally and they sought means to convince him. Support of their views by some influential male would help but this was not easy to obtain.

E.G. to E.D.   *Bayswater, 4 July 1860*

'Mr. and Mrs. Gurney were extremely kind and helpful this morning and we have found some one who can be relied upon to give Father a strongly favourable opinion of the movement. You remember a Mr. Hawes whom Miss Blackwell[1] mentioned. This morning Mr. Gurney spoke of William Hawes and I found that this Mr. Hawes is the same that my father knows very well. They did a great deal of business together a few years ago and I am pretty sure that his opinion will have weight. Mr. Gurney kindly proposed asking him to meet me at their house, before we send my father to him. Mr. Gurney also offered to see my father and tell him *his* opinion, which I thought extremely kind.'

Mr. Hawes advised Elizabeth to go into a surgical ward at the Middlesex Hospital for a preliminary period of six months. He could arrange this, he said. It was to test her resolution that Mr. Hawes suggested a surgical ward where conditions at that time, even in the best hospitals, were bad. Mr. Hawes knew that the sights, sounds and smells in a surgical ward would provide a searching test. In 1860 bacteriology was in its infancy and the connection between living germs and wound infection had occurred to no one. The mortality after major operations was appalling, and even in trivial cases infection might occur. It was not unusual for surgeons to demonstrate in the dissecting-room, conduct a post-mortem examination or dress a gangrenous wound, and then to operate.

For ward visits a frock-coat was worn and for the

[1] Elizabeth sometimes gives but often omits the professional title.

coat's sake it was exchanged for an old one before the surgeon entered the theatre. Usually he washed his hands after operating, not necessarily before. Gloves were not worn. Sterilization of ligatures and instruments was unknown. A favourite dressing, if not the poultice, was lint teased by convalescent patients. The suppuration of wounds was expected and great was the relief of the surgeon when it could be described as 'laudable pus'. Hospital gangrene often led to the temporary closure of wards. Under these conditions, surgery was at a discount. Few operations were done and they consisted largely of the amputation of limbs for compound fractures. Then came the great advance. Joseph Lister, pondering over Pasteur's germ theory, proclaimed himself his disciple. He was certain that inflammation and suppuration of wounds were caused by the introduction of living germs. By 1867 Lister had evolved his method. 'Listerism' was the name at first given but later it became known as the antiseptic system of surgery. Lister taught that when the protection of the skin is removed by cut or injury, the tissues are at the mercy of germs conveyed by the air or more often by the surgeon himself. He wrote to Pasteur, 13 February 1874: 'I do not know if the records of British surgery ever meet your eye. If so, you will have seen from time to time notices of the antiseptic system of treatment which I have been labouring for the last nine years to bring to perfection. Allow me to take this opportunity to tender you my most cordial thanks for having, by your brilliant researches, demonstrated to me the truth of the germ theory of putrefaction and thus furnished me with the principle upon which alone the antiseptic system can be carried out.' [*Life of Pasteur* by R. Vallory-Radot.]

Every innovation is opposed, but in spite of hostility and ridicule, Lister gradually transformed surgical procedure and the era of modern surgery began. The carbolic spray in the theatre soaked those present, while bowls of pungent lotion reminded the surgeon and his assistants of the care they had to take. A tribute has been paid to Lister recently by Sir St. Clair Thomson, who was his house surgeon in 1883. He described Lister as 'the greatest of all masters of surgery', and said that the application of his principles even during his lifetime saved more lives than all the wars of Napoleon had destroyed. 'Before Lister's time', Sir St. Clair Thomson said, 'surgery was accompanied by great horrors. The causes of sepsis were not then known. Even the most trifling wound might become septic or a pin-prick might be the door to death. The operation death-rate before the coming of Lister and even in his own wards in early days was from 25 to 40 per cent. The chances were that one out of every three or four patients operated on would die. Sometimes in military hospitals the death-rate would mount to 75 or 90 per cent. Erichsen, to whom Lister had been house-surgeon, prophesied in 1874 that 'the abdomen, chest and brain would be for ever shut from the intrusion of the wise and humane surgeon,' while another surgeon had pronounced that 'an abdominal operation should be classed amongst the methods of the executioner.' [*British Medical Journal*, 15 October 1938, Sir St. Clair Thomson, University College Med. Sch., 11 October 1938.] The lament of Nelaton, the French surgeon, is recorded in *The Life of Pasteur*. During the siege of Paris 1870, 'Nelaton in despair at the death of almost every patient who had been operated on, declared that he who should conquer purulent infection would deserve a golden statue.'

Elizabeth went to the Middlesex Hospital before Lister's principles had been evolved.

E.G. to E.D.   *Bayswater, 8 July 1860*

'Mr. Hawes was cordial enough yesterday morning. He asked me if I had any idea of the nature of these difficulties, and when I said that it was because I felt so ignorant about them, that I dared not speak or think confidently of the strength of my determination, he suggested that some test should be found to prove my power of endurance &c. *before* any time was spent upon direct medical studies. I thought this very reasonable, if there really are such great unknown difficulties, and as Mr. and Mrs. Gurney seemed to agree with Mr. Hawes on this point, I suggested that I should spend 6 months as hospital nurse at once, as a test. I shall of course go to the hospital to-morrow.'

Medical Training

Elizabeth was never dilatory. A letter from her father, received the same day, pleased her. It was characteristic and generous.

N.G. to E.G.   *Aldeburgh, 8 July 1860*

'I have resolved in my own mind after deep and painful consideration not to oppose your wishes and views and as far as expense is involved I will do all I can, in justice to my other children, to assist you in your study. As far as I am able to judge, the plan of going into a woman's ward in one of the London hospitals as a nurse is the best, but here again I say I feel myself so totally unable to advise. Your dear mother is very anxious on this subject.'

Preliminary arrangements were made with Mr. de Morgan, the hospital treasurer, and, as Elizabeth felt her plans were taking shape, she started to break the news to friends and relations.

E.G. to E.D.   *Bayswater, 11 July 1860*

'You will be pleased to see my father's note, as it is quite as cordial a sanction as we could hope he would give. I called upon Mrs. Gurney this morning to tell her what arrangements I had made for the future, and to say good-bye. She was exceedingly kind, almost dangerously so, for I grew afraid that a touch more of tenderness would make me cry. I have been paying a round of family calls this morning, for the express purpose of telling my intentions to those who must hear of them

very soon. I think we prospered very well. Every one
was very much startled at first, but they all came round
to a very cordial agreement as to the desirableness of
women having something to do, and as to the propriety
of medicine being studied by women. I am heartily
ashamed of this very inelegant sentence.'

Perhaps Elizabeth took special trouble over her letter
to Mrs. Richard Garrett, at any rate she kept a copy of
it.

E.G. to Mrs. Richard Garrett   Aldeburgh, 13 July 1860
'For some time I have been gradually making up my
mind to an important step, and now that the time for
action has come, I do not like to take it without telling
my friends what I am about to do. During the last two
or three years, I have felt an increasing longing for some
definite occupation, which should also bring me, in
time, a position and moderate income. I think you will
not be surprised that I should feel this longing for it is
indeed far more wonderful that a healthy woman should
spend a long life in comparative idleness than that she
should wish for some suitable work, upon which she
could spend the energy that now only causes painful
restlessness and weariness. I have decided that the study
of medicine offers more attractions to me than any other
kind of work, and I have resolved to enter upon it. It is
generally admitted that there would be no impropriety
in women and children being attended by physicians of

their own sex, and it is these branches of the profession which we wish to see opened to women. For this reason, I have arranged to spend six months in the Middlesex Hospital as a nurse, as I have been assured by those who are qualified to judge, that this will be a sufficiently searching test. I need scarcely say that I should not make this attempt without my dear parents' sanction. Whatever the issue of the attempt may be, I shall always remember their sympathy and consideration with gratitude.'

    E.G. to E.D.   *Aldeburgh, 16 July 1860*
  'I am glad to say that though I grow tired of talking about myself the more I think about my scheme the more do I like it. It would be a great disappointment now to have to abandon it.'

    E.G. to E.D.   *Aldeburgh, 19 July 1860*
  'Every one seems to fear that my health and nerves will break down. Therefore I am determined by God's help to keep in good health, if care can do it. I had a long letter from William Freeman [husband of Elizabeth's cousin Sarah] yesterday exhorting me to abandon the attempt and another from my Aunt Rd. [Mrs. Richard Garrett] this morning to the same effect. I was very careful not to imply (in writing to inform my friends of my intention) that I wanted their advice, this caution has been useless however, for they all seem to think it necessary to give me a most liberal dose of it, and when

Medical Training

I cannot follow it there is some awkwardness in thanking them for their kind solicitude.'

In August Elizabeth went to London to start work. It was arranged that she should live, as far as possible, with her sister Louie, then at 7 St. Agnes Villas, Bayswater.

Every institution creates its own atmosphere and into the small world of the Middlesex Hospital Elizabeth entered on 1st August 1860, alert and grave, thrilled and circumspect. She provided herself with a linen apron and a note-book. At the end of a week she wrote as though she were a senior student. She met with consideration and kindness. Mrs. Yarrow, the matron, set the tone among the nurses, and they welcomed the newcomer and taught her how to dress wounds and to care for sick people. The senior resident medical officer, Mr. Willis, was ready to discuss her future and to demonstrate clinical signs. Mr. Nunn, the dean and assistant surgeon, was cordial; he had charge of the dissecting-room in addition to his work in the operating theatre, an arrangement which throws light on the practice of a good general hospital at that date. T. W. Nunn, known affectionately as Tommy to the entire hospital, was a most popular dean from 1859 to 1867.

E.G. to E.D.   *Bayswater, 7 Aug. 1860*
'I think as I go on, I shall constantly feel my way into *more* work in the hospital, so that what I give as my round of duties now will probably not continue exactly

true for many days to come. I get to the hospital by
8 a.m. and as I am now familiar with the different cases
in the 2 surgical wards in which I am located, I begin at
once to prepare for the dressings by spreading the different ointments, preparing lint, lotion, poultices, bandages
&c. While I am doing this at a side table, the sister is
going round and examining all wounds &c. The simpler
cases she leaves entirely to me very often, but the more
difficult ones, such as cancer, she dresses herself while I
look on. If I can manage to be in the medical wards with
the house doctor and then return to the surgical cases in
time for the surgeon's visit I like to do so. The doctors
are uncommonly civil to me from the house-surgeon
upwards. There was a small operation in the ward to-
day, which I saw, and the surgeon was very kind in
explaining the case to me, and making me see what he
was going to do. There was only one pupil with him,
but he made him stand out of my way and took special
care of my situation &c. Mr. Worthington, the house-
surgeon, is also very courteous in giving me information.
This afternoon, Mr. Nunn, the surgeon who had done
the small operation, asked me if I should like to go to
the out-patient department, and when I said that I
should, he promised to take me there in a week or two,
when he returns from the country. There is a great deal
more to tell you—verily I cannot go on much longer. I
wish one could write more quickly. My father was here
last night, and seemed in good spirits, and interested in

all my details.' She added: 'Writing is a great treat and rest, besides being sometimes a duty.'

The next letter to Miss Davies reported that Mrs. Garrett was suffering from a relapse of depression.

E.G. to E.D.   *Bayswater, 17 Aug. 1860*

'I have been a good deal perplexed by receiving most melancholy letters from home, and about my mother. It appears as if she had suddenly made up her mind that I had acted in a most wilful manner, and in opposition to her earnest request, which is, of course, a purely imaginary state of things; she speaks of my step being a source of life-long pain to her, that it is a living death, etc., indeed her tone was alarmingly morbid throughout. By the same post I had several letters from anxious relatives, telling me that it was my duty to come home and thus ease my mother's anxiety. I think this is quite stupid advice. At any rate, I think every other means should be used before this be tried. I am very much in hopes that a very much more cheerful view will be taken of me in a few weeks. I am getting on very well professionally—does not that sound sweet? The pupils too seem inclined to treat me as a student and as long as they merely speak to me of the matter in hand, I think it is wiser not to appear too frigid and stiff with them. If they *will* forget my sex and treat me as a fellow student, it is just the right kind of feeling. It does seem to be wrong in theory to treat them all as one's natural enemies, though

I know that in practice an absence of stiffness might be misconstrued.'

From the day she started work at the hospital, Elizabeth determined to avoid gossip; she would be closely watched, even friendliness might be criticized. To treat the staff as strangers when the majority were cordial and considerate must have been an effort, but she did not relax until later, with Mr. Nunn and the invaluable Mr. Plaskitt, whose help will be recorded presently. Elizabeth's view of herself was humble; she thought she had no charm, for men at any rate, and that she was plain; but charm or no charm she eased her path by making friends with the people she worked with, and among the medical staff at the Middlesex she made lasting friendships.

E.G. to E.D.　　　　　　　　　*Bayswater, 5 Sept. 1860*
'I had some talk with Dr. Willis a few days ago. He is very kind in giving me a good deal of information, and if he should continue at the hospital I don't think I could do better than by asking him to take me as a pupil. I don't find that it makes any difference whether the doctors are young or old, or married or single, as far as being taught by them goes. Dr. Willis takes everything so calmly that I do not feel half as much awkwardness with what he says to me and shows me, as I do with the hesitation and would-be modesty of some of the old physicians. I am almost forgetting to tell you that I went

through my first operation yesterday. It was a stiffish one, and I did not feel at all bad, the excitement was very great but happily it took the form of quickening all my vitality, instead of depressing it. Experience is modifying my notions about the most suitable style of dress for me to wear at the hospital. I feel confident now that one is helped rather than hindered by being as much like a lady as lies in one's power. When my student life begins, I shall try to get very serviceable, rich, whole coloured dresses that will do without trimmings and not require renewing often. Miss A. Leigh Smith came into the luncheon-room yesterday as I was fortifying myself with a mutton chop and ale, and gave me some fresh spirit as a look at her face generally does.'

Miss Davies felt the importance of being a 'lady-like lady' and Elizabeth agreed with her. The work was engrossing, but to be thrust into the wards before she had mastered preliminary subjects made understanding difficult. Much that the doctors said was incomprehensible. She lamented her ignorance of Greek, as many medical terms were taken directly from it. In September she moved into lodgings in South Audley Street, with Miss Sarah Smith, sister of her brother-in-law James Smith, as chaperon. A day in the country [Acton] gave her great pleasure.

E.G. to E.D.   *S. Audley St., 9 Sept. 1860*
'I went to Acton yesterday, and came home about an

hour ago. I have enjoyed the day in the country excessively. The cornfields are so beautiful. I will send you a
full prospectus of the Middlesex Hospital Medical College, as I think you will like to look over it. I wrote
formally to the Dean for it and it was sent at once. I will
also send a note received from Mr. Hawes. As he knows
several members of the Governing Board, I thought it
would be well to remind him of my existence and sus-
tain his interest, by writing to tell him how I was getting
on. It is rather provoking that people will think so much
of the difficulties, in spite of my assurances that so far
from their being appalling I am enjoying the work more
than I have ever done any other study or pursuit. Sometimes I fear I must be dreadfully obtuse, not to feel what
every one seems to think must be so trying, but if this is
the case, I can only accept it as a fact and make the best
of it. I am very sorry not to be more sensitive in some
other things, but it is difficult to see how to increase a
power of this kind, which is almost essentially a birth-
right.'

She was given a room at the hospital but her irregular
position troubled her. She wanted to pay fees like an
ordinary student.

E.G. to E.D.   *Middlesex Hospital, 29 Sept. 1860*
'Your two letters reached me together last night. I sat
over the fire and enjoyed them very much. The room
has all cottage peculiarities and having to set out my own

meals harmonizes with its aspect. One of the nurses is good enough to cook for me, and they would all willingly do more if I did not wish to try my hand at the sister's work just as it is. I have done the linen for the wash, taken the medicine to the shop, and brought up stores from the housekeeper this morning, in addition to the proper nursing work. The doctors who are most civil to me now are not those who will have anything to do with admitting me as a student, with the one valuable exception of Mr. Nunn, in whom I place a good deal of confidence. He has asked me to dine with him as soon as his wife comes back to London that we may discuss my plans. He is evidently very fond of teaching and goes out of his way to do so pretty often. I should like to know a good deal more of the Drewrys, superior people are so very valuable. I think one would be justified in giving up time for their acquaintance. I should be very glad to have Ellen Drewry as a fellow student. I have come to the conclusion that it will not do to go on long in the false position I now occupy at the hospital. I have accordingly written to Mr. De Morgan, the treasurer of the college, asking to see him when next he comes to the hospital, and I shall know much more of the chance of being admitted as a student when he gives his opinion upon this proposal. If the medical board are determined never to admit me I should have to recast all my plans.'

Medical Training

In the next letter Elizabeth explained her duties as a night nurse.

E.G. to Jane Crowe   Middlesex Hospital, 9 Oct. 1860
'I am now on night duty, this is the first night, and I am in a medical ward with a good many helpless patients. I am sitting by the fire, with screens round and gas light within, but of course I must listen and go round the ward pretty often. Mr. De Morgan met me last Monday and we went into the question [of admission as a student]. I had chosen to consult him rather than Mr. Nunn who is Dean and has equal power, as I knew the latter would help me and Mr. De Morgan might be brought round by personal influence. The result was not quite as satisfactory as I could have wished, but there is a fair proportion of favourable things to tell you. He would not allow me to pay any fees as that would be recognizing me partially as a student but I may make a donation to the hospital and stay through the winter learning all I can as an amateur. I may also continue in the surgery as long as I like and attend the house doctors in their rounds, and go to operations and have the run of the house as at present. The Board has also given me the temporary use of a very pleasant room in which I can read and keep my things. This is a great comfort and will save no end of time. Mr. de Morgan said that the apothecary could take me as a pupil if he likes to do so. As soon as Mr. De Morgan left, I saw Mr. Plaskitt the

apothecary, and found him very willing to take me, so
I have settled to go to him for 3 or 4 hours daily for 6
months, beginning in a fortnight's time. It is something
to gain this footing in even one department, though Mr.
De Morgan was very discouraging about the ultimate
chance of getting into the college. He said it was impossible, but would not assign any grounds for such an
opinion except that a lady's presence at lectures would
distract the other students' attention. All that he said
against it was as frivolous as this is, and on the whole I
did not feel hopeful about ever bringing him round, he
was too much inclined to treat the subject with amused
contempt. He thinks all the London colleges will refuse
to admit me, and that I might as well go to America at
once. I shall use every effort however to get the education in England and in the regular way though I believe
much may be done irregularly. I shall do the dissecting
work in my room here, to spare Louie's nerves and
myself the trouble of carrying the pieces to and fro.'

Mr. Joshua Plaskitt had been resident medical officer
at the Middlesex Hospital. Although not a member of
the honorary medical staff, his position as apothecary-
dispenser brought him to the hospital constantly. His
interest in the solitary student grew to friendship and his
help was to prove invaluable. He was cultured and liberal-
minded and elsewhere Elizabeth reported that although
young he was not 'flighty' and she thought 'safe'.

Medical Training

Another letter written in the ward behind the screen while on night duty was less cheerful. Miss Drewry's clothes and perhaps the hour [4 a.m.] had a depressing effect apart from more important difficulties.

E.G. to E.D.   Middlesex Hp. 4 a.m., 12 Oct. 1860

'Miss E. Drewry and I have arranged to study chemistry together. I believe that a fellow student of wit will be more help to me than a master would be. I do wish that the Drewrys dressed better. After the arrangement was made for her to come here I was almost afraid it was unwise on my part. She looks awfully strong-minded in walking dress but as my room is out of the way I hope she will not be supposed to belong to me by the students, etc. She has short petticoats and a close round hat and several other dreadfully ugly arrangements: it is a serious mistake I think for a respectable woman to fall into. Do you ever feel wearied with your own want of power? The sense of it comes to me constantly now, if I were given a much larger measure so much more could be done in every way with the opportunities here. It is hard to be contented with a gooseberry nature, when one sees that a peach is wanted.'

At this period Elizabeth's letters contain constant references to the Rev. F. D. Maurice who accepted the incumbency of Vere Street Chapel in 1860. Elizabeth was a regular member of the congregation, and his broad-minded theology, and interest in social problems and sympathy with many aspects of the women's movement made his sermons inspiring to her. Mr. Maurice had founded the Working Men's College, and in 1848 Queen's College for Women in Harley Street, the object of the latter being to supply 'female knowledge to governesses', i.e. suitable information on general education to women. To the surprise and regret of some of his followers, Mr. Maurice disapproved of teaching women biology and still more was he opposed to training women for the medical profession. Thus it came about that while he uplifted the spirit of Elizabeth Garrett, he kept himself remote from her and perhaps never spoke to her, certainly never asked her to his house.

She continued to send Emily notes of sermons partly as a literary exercise.

E.G. to E.D.   *Middlesex Hp., 14 Oct. 1860*
'Mr. Maurice's sermon was very fine this morning. I have written a few notes of what I can remember of it. They naturally look much less striking than the spoken words were. Thanks to my friendly spectacles I discovered Mr. Nunn among the congregation. We met on leaving and he introduced me to Mrs. Nunn and I went home with them. When we reached their house I asked when I could have some conversation with him and he said "at once" so we went in and had a very cheering discussion for half an hour. Mr. Nunn was so encouraging that I was emboldened to ask him to take me as a private

pupil. He said he would, but I do not consider it settled yet as I thought he ought to think about it before deciding, though it is pretty clear from his manner that he would not refuse to help because I am a woman as Mr. De Morgan hinted he should. He asked me how old I was, and was very much surprised to hear that I was more than 18.'

Many girls would have read a compliment into these words: not so Elizabeth, who was incapable of the mildest coquetry. It was as well; to have suspected Mr. Nunn of approaching the confines of 'flightiness' would have shocked her. He possessed a sitting in Christ Church and a wife, both bulwarks against such a failing. Also, she respected him and placed 'considerable confidence' in him. The letter continues, 'Dr. Willis has just been in for his night visit. He says a tutor would be of great use to me to examine me thoroughly in my reading. How would it do to ask Dr. Willis to come to Manchester Square one evening (or 2, if he could) and act as tutor? I should not think he would be annoyed at my asking, at least, as it is not very unusual for people to take pupils. I think he is a safe person both as to right feeling and sound education, but I should not like to set my friends or the people here gossiping and you cannot trust to their understanding it simply. Please tell me what you think.'

Miss Davies, the most cautious of reformers, wrote to advise Elizabeth against asking Mr. Willis to coach her.

Medical Training

She thought propriety mattered more than the teaching. Meantime he had offered to do so and, supported by her parents and Louie, this kind suggestion had been accepted.

E.G. to E.D.   *South Audley St., 23 Oct. 1860*

'Your advice about Dr. Willis has come too late to take any but a negative effect. The last night that I sat up at the hospital, he asked me if he could be of any use as a tutor. He offered to come to my house three nights a week, for 2 hours, and the terms would be a guinea a week. Though I had been thinking of asking him to do this, it was somewhat perplexing to have to decide if it would really be right and wise. I felt sure about its being a great help to me as he has a clear method of explaining and does look at things in the professional unawkward way. On the other hand there was one's reputation and the chance of losing anything in this direction. I thought the whole thing over during that night, and wrote to my father for his views. Miss Annie Leigh Smith and Miss Blythe called the next morning to my great enjoyment. I told them of the proposal and though Miss Smith saw the difficulties she was in favour of risking these for the sake of the teaching. My parents and Louie took the same view, so I have accepted the offer, and as soon as we go to Manchester Square [the Smiths' new house] the lessons will begin. The vulgarity of other people is the difficulty, it is so impossible to forget that to many, simple and honest actions will seem wonderful and wrong. I consider my engagement with Mr. Plaskitt is some safeguard in this respect, it looks well to be taught by several doctors at once, and the sisters and nurses will know of this even more surely than they will of Dr. Willis' lessons. Mr. Plaskitt is young, but so very quiet and unflighty that no one would say anything in connection with him, and he will serve as a shield, I hope. Your advice will make me more than ever cautious, though I cannot act positively upon it. My father is very kind and liberal, now that I have started he wishes me to spare no expense and to make any arrangements I may think best. He thinks Dr. Willis' charge very little. Mr. Plaskitt expects me to know a great deal more than I do and makes me parse Latin to him whenever there is a stiff piece in the Pharmacopœia.'

At the end of October Louie and James Smith moved from Bayswater to Manchester Square where Elizabeth joined them. It was a larger house and near the Middlesex Hospital.

E.G. to E.D.   *Manchester Square, 30 Oct. 1860*
'You shall have one of the first letters from the new house. Dr. Willis has been this evening for the first lesson and it went off very comfortably and with no awkwardness. Dr. Willis has given me plenty to do for the next lesson so that with Mr. Plaskitt, Miss Drewry and hospital attendance, I shall be fully employed. I do no

nursing now, but merely go into the wards to watch the cases. To-day I was nearly faint from want of food as he [Mr. Plaskitt] made me go on reading Latin to him till 3 o'clock though I had protested at 2 that I was very hungry.'

Louie's house provided constant hospitality for the family, who enjoyed being together. Even so, Elizabeth had to admit that as the third person and permanent visitor in the Smith household her chances of showing hospitality to her own friends were limited. She regretted this as her instincts were sociable. The Rev. J. Llewelyn Davies, Rector of Christ Church, Marylebone, the friend and disciple of Mr. Maurice, was a staunch supporter of the women's movement. His services were attended and reported to his sister Emily. Throughout life, he was to be an active and stimulating friend to medical women, especially to Elizabeth.

E.G. to E.D.   *Manchester Square, 12 Dec. 1860*
'Mr. Plaskitt and Dr. Willis are going to give me examination papers to-morrow week on their several subjects, as I wished for some kind of test to see how clear my general conceptions are. Mr. Plaskitt says I should be locked up in an empty room, but if I deliver up all books to him he will leave me free. Sometimes I feel very much dissatisfied with myself, though I have always known that my powers were of the kind to make success difficult. I am not sure that the cause will be

injured by this, so that it ought not to be any weight upon one. Probably as the majority of women are not much more gifted than I am, an example from one of their own calibre will be more useful than from a more brilliant person, though on other grounds one would wish the success to be as undoubted as probably only a gifted woman could make it. There is so much to say to you now that a letter is started. Jane Crowe told us of the Working Men's College Rifle Corps going to Christ Church so Agnes and I hurried away from dinner and by the aid of a hansom reached the church as soon as the Corps did. The congregation was very grand. I do enjoy a crowd excessively, and it is as fine in a church as anywhere, I think. I was delighted with the improvement in the singing. The sermon was especially clear and interesting and directly upon the rifle corps subject, if there is any time after this letter is finished I will put down some of it for you. We met Mr. Davies [the Rector] after the service. Agnes was very much struck with his face, she thinks it is like the pictures of our Saviour.'

After five months away from home Elizabeth found Christmas at Aldeburgh pleasant. 'There is something inexplicably delightful in coming back to familiar places and things.' She felt certain that her absence from home had done no harm. 'In truth I cannot see that the smallest degree of mischief has been done here by my move.' The holiday was brief and soon she was back at the hospital.

Medical Training

Although she worked hard some relaxation was permitted. Mrs. Davies gave an evening party and Elizabeth was privileged to stand near the Rev. F. D. Maurice and to hear his conversation with Mrs. Russell Gurney.

E.G. to E.D.   Middlesex Hospital, 16 Feb. 1861
'I enjoyed Mrs. Davies' party very much, seeing Mr. Maurice in some kind of private life was very pleasant. He and Mrs. Gurney talked together for some time and I stood as near as I could and took in the sight and sounds to my heart's content. There was nothing particularly interesting talked about, I think, the party was too large for that, but perhaps it is the sociable, less earnest side [in Mr. Maurice] one chiefly wishes to see after being familiar with the other in books and sermons. Mr. Hughes was talking a great deal about the Rifle Corps and its officers.'

The temporary arrangement by which Elizabeth had the use of a room at the hospital in which she could dissect had come to an end. She greatly hoped that Mr. Nunn would introduce her into the students' dissecting-room as the alternative—carrying 'bits' to and from her sister's house to dissect in her bedroom was not attractive. Meanwhile it was consoling to discover a fellow student, in his second year, who did not even know the healthy heart sounds. Physicians and surgeons at this time were obliged to make their diagnoses on the results of infinitely careful observations. No X-ray photograph could be demanded and no test meals given. Blood examinations were of the simplest, biochemistry did not exist.

E.G. to E.D.   *Manchester Square, 6 March 1861*

'Thanks for your letter. I have been waiting to send Miss Blackwell's letter, but it is still at Aldeburgh. My father was very much pleased with it. Miss B's advice has modified my more immediate plans a little, I mean to try for entrance into the dissecting-room as soon as I am ready to work there and postpone raising the question of admittance perhaps for another year. Mr. Nunn has the control of the dissecting-room, so I hope it will be possible to get there; and next winter session I shall try for admittance to the chemical lectures and laboratory, which will be the small end of the wedge for the lectures generally. I am studying nearly the whole day now, as the lessons with Mr. Plaskitt are pausing, in consequence of the floor of his room being up and my refusal to read Tacitus standing on a plank. I am glad to have some extra time to grind away at anatomy. I want to be ready for the dissecting-room by May when the summer session will begin.'

About this time Mr. Plaskitt announced that he was leaving the hospital to go into general practice as a member of a medical firm. This was bad news for Elizabeth but through Mr. Nunn's recommendation she was invited to attend the lectures of Mr. Taylor on chemistry, and at last she entered the dissecting-room to find it less trying than she had expected.

E.G. to E.D.   *22 Manchester Sq., 12 April 1861*
'Dr. Willis has just left and I feel able to enjoy putting anatomy away for the night. We finished the arteries to-night and now thank Heaven only the veins and nerves remain. I go round with Dr. Thompson now. He is a Fellow of St. John's, Cambridge, and an examiner at the College of Physicians, it is very difficult to catch what he is talking about. However he is very civil, and knowledge is a secondary thing till I have broken down the opposition of those who will have the power of keeping me out of the School. I feel so mean in trying to come over the doctors by all kinds of little feminine dodges but Mrs. Gurney seemed to think they did not matter. She said it was often a matter of perplexity to her to know if feminine arts were lawful in a good cause. She thinks they have immense weight from any woman. I can believe her own to be very powerful.'

In May 1861 Elizabeth was accepted for some special courses of lectures and demonstrations and for these she paid fees, but Mr. de Morgan would not allow her to enter as a regular student for the whole course. She went to practical chemistry demonstrations and noted that, 'I have had to sign my name in the College books in token that I will not smoke but will in every way comport myself as a gentleman.'

77

Medical Training

Elizabeth kept in touch with Dr. Elizabeth Blackwell, and after telling her of the work at the hospital asked her opinion 'upon the plan of applying for admittance as a student for the next winter session and also what you would advise in the event of this being refused.'

E.G. to E.D.   *Manchester Square, 6 May 1861*

'I determined to ask Dr. Thompson to admit me to his lectures [on materia medica]. It being the opening day of the session he had an unusual train of pupils, and for some time I thought it must be put off till another day. However this seemed cowardly, and moreover as the course had begun any delay was injurious, so I screwed up my courage and asked him as he was leaving the ward. Dr. Thompson looked confounded with my boldness and before he answered I told him that the Chemical Professors had admitted me to their classes; this settled his doubts and he said very cordially that he should be glad to see me. I felt tremendously triumphant, tho' it was not so much after all. The next day I avoided him carefully fearing he might have repented, and to-day I have been to his lecture and the Practical Chemistry. I have had business interviews with Mr. De Morgan (who promised to vote against me last autumn) and Mr. Nunn, and they were both encouraging. Mr. De Morgan took the lecture fees and put me down on the books as a student. He is much more friendly than he was, and I hope he would not oppose me now. I told

78

him I wanted to be admitted fully in October, but had
no intention of asking this formally till he and a decided
majority of the committee showed themselves really
willing to receive me. I thought of Mrs. Gurney and
feminine arts, with a longing to work him round somehow. He asked if I were going in for prizes, forgetting
(or pretending to do so) that these can only be got by
those who attend all the lectures of the session, but when
I reminded him of this, he said, "But at least you may
get a certificate of honour, for each separate course of
lectures." While I was in the Board Room to-day with
Mr. Nunn, Dr. Stewart [senior physician] came in, and
presently came to me, and said that if I still wished to
go round with him, he should have much pleasure in
my doing so. He is a horribly unpunctual man, seldom
coming till an hour and half after his time, but of course
I accepted his offer, and went with him to-day. He can
be heard, and is a good doctor.'

As the months passed, Elizabeth grew more confident,
perhaps over-confident, about her position at the hospital. To have the dean on her side anxious to help gave
her a sense of security. In June 1861 however she began to
be dissatisfied with her progress at the hospital. Mr. Nunn
had withdrawn or modified his consent about the dissecting-room; perhaps pressure had been put on him by other
members of the medical committee. Also she noticed less
cordiality in the manner of the out-patient physician.

Medical Training

E.G. to E.D.   *Manchester Square, 4 June 1861*

'I am not satisfied with my progress with the physicians, especially with Dr. Murchison, whose out-patients I see. He is certainly growing less civil than he was at first, and I can't account for it at all, unless it is that he does not like to see me pushing into the lectures and other student privileges.'

Elizabeth obtained a certificate of honour in each class examination; she did so well indeed that the examiner in sending her the list added, 'May I entreat you to use every precaution in keeping this a secret from the students?' In June trouble arose. The visiting physician asked his class a question, none of the men could answer and Elizabeth gave the right reply. The students were angry and petitioned for her dismissal. A counter-petition was sent to the committee but she was told that she would be admitted to no more lectures although she might finish those for which she had paid fees.

E.G. to E.D.   *Manchester Square, 7 June 1861*

'Jane [Crowe] told me that she mentioned to you about the wretched memorial against me. I could not settle down to doing nothing, and so wrote to the students. At first I thought of leaving the letter in their room, but then it occurred to me that perhaps some ill-disposed student might see it first and quietly keep it from the others. So I wrote to Mr. Fowler, Mr. Plaskitt's successor, and asked him to give the letter to the leader of the

movement. The answer has come to-night. They will
not give up the memorial, but I don't mind so much,
now that I know there is as strong a division for me as
against me. Mr. Plaskitt called on me to-day and told
me many of the good ones were standing up against the
memorial like bricks, he found one of the medical assistants whom I had never known as a friend, defending
me and pitching into the memorial with a flushed face
and an air of great annoyance, so, on the whole, it perhaps may do as much good as harm, though I fear some
of the lecturers who are still against me will make the
memorial a handle for their own prejudices: I felt horribly crushed yesterday, it was so bad to think all the
way gained during this year was to be lost in that way.'

This is her letter to the students:

Draft letter to the students from E.G. (undated)
'Gentlemen. Will you pardon me for addressing a few
lines to you on the subject of my admission as a student
into the Medical School of this Hospital. I have heard
to-day of your decision to memorialize the lecturers
against the admission of women students. The personal
courtesy I have always received from you makes me
venture upon the unusual step of begging you to recon-
sider that decision or at least to delay for a time sending
up the memorial. I am fully aware of the weight such a
memorial would justly have with the lecturers, and this
request to delay it, arises from a fear on my part, lest you

should use your power somewhat cruelly from not recognizing its extent. If my presence would really prevent the lecturers from giving their usual course of instruction, you would have a right—that of possession at least—to object to any change followed by such a result. But surely if the lecturers would guarantee that there should be no change whatever in their lectures, all legitimate ground of objection would be removed. In conclusion I would submit that this question is of far greater importance to me than to any fellow student. I *may* unwillingly make you lose some teaching, you certainly can shut me out from all.'

E.G. to E.D.   *Manchester Square, 11 June 1861*
'Condole with me! I believe my death-warrant will be signed next Thursday, as far as the Middlesex people can do it. It is horribly vexing but I don't despair, trials are good and I very seldom have any, and it won't stop me from studying nor from finally doing my work whatever that may be. We are apt to make mistakes about vocations, but I suppose we may rest in the belief that God will keep us in His Service somehow if we try to see what and where it is, with open minds. I do not feel at all crushed, though somewhat adrift. I had made up my mind to getting in here and going through the business with an air of graceful ease. The Chemical Class will be examined to-morrow morning. Mr. Heisch, the lecturer, half advised me not to be present, as the students

will be left alone to write their papers and make experiments, but as I mentioned the examinations expressly at the time I paid the fees, I will not be frightened out of them. The students dare not be rude, I am sure, and if they were, I should survive it. I suppose you will be too tired to come down *here* to-morrow night and hear the result? However do please come to the hospital on Thursday at six o'clock, we could have tea together and go to the Bach Society's private performance of the Christmas Oratorio afterwards; as my fate will then be sealed, I shall be able to listen.'

The friendly students wrote to Elizabeth.

Students to E.G.   Middlesex Hospital, 12 June 1861
'We, the undersigned students of this Hospital, desire to express our regret at the part taken by some of our fellow students in framing and sending in a Memorial to the Medical Committee respecting your attendance at lectures, etc. We beg to intimate that the substance of that Memorial is not an expression of the sentiments of the whole of the students of this School of Medicine.'

To this letter there were five signatures.

Draft letter E.G. to friendly students
                    Middlesex Hospital (undated)
'Gentlemen. I am quite unable to thank you adequately for your kind and generous letter. Believe me, it will be remembered most gratefully long after the Memorial

and its promoters are forgotten. Will you permit me to add, that whatever may be the issue of to-morrow's decision regarding myself, I shall always feel rejoiced to hear of your success and advancement.'

E.G. to E.D.   *Middlesex Hospital, 14 June 1861*

'The meeting was not adjourned yesterday as we hoped from not hearing the result, the fact is, the decision was so disagreeable that Mr. Nunn and my other friends did not like to come and tell me. I asked Dr. Thompson this morning and he brought it out very nervously, as if he feared I should go off into hysterics or embarrass him in some way. The reasons they give are, the lecturers dislike the presence of women, and that the school would suffer. The lecturers regretted that this decision had been arrived at "in the case of a lady whose conduct had, during her entire stay in the hospital, been marked by a union of judgment and delicacy which had commanded their entire esteem".'

Mrs. Gurney shared the disappointment of all Elizabeth's friends. The support Mr. Russell Gurney and she gave to the advancement of women made their friendship invaluable.

Mrs. Gurney to E.G.   *Palace Gardens (undated)*

'No, dear Miss Garrett, we will not, we *cannot* pity you because you have a spirit which places you above all circumstances. The manner in which you have acted makes us respect and admire you the more—but we cannot help grieving for the *cause*, which must suffer so much if you are baffled.'

The *Lancet* published an unfriendly article to which Mr. Plaskitt referred when he wrote about her proposal to be bound in apprenticeship to him.

Mr. Plaskitt to E.G.   *Chapel St., 16 June 1861*

'It would be easy to find some one to whom you could be bound 'prentice in the merely nominal way the [Apothecaries'] Hall is satisfied with. You do me the honour to select me as the person to whom you should bear that relation, and now that I have recovered from the amusement which the strangeness of the proposal at first gave me, I am to tell you seriously and "frankly" what I have to say in reply. As far, then, as I myself am concerned I should not have the faintest objection to enter into an agreement with you of the kind sketched out in your note, but I think my part in a transaction of this nature might possibly affect me as a member of a business firm, and, therefore, that the question ought first to be submitted to those with whom in all matters of business I am bound up. This done, and their approval obtained (for I do not anticipate objection), I shall be happy to return to the subject, and, should you still be in the same mind, arrange details. I have a note to write to Mrs. Smith about a strawberry feast to which she has invited me at Acton. I shall go, if possible. I have seen and read the article in the *Lancet* since receiving your note. I fear it will add to your embarrassment. The circumstance as then alluded to is calculated to create a totally different impression from what would arise if the *whole* truth were told. With respect to the expediency of answering the article, do you think it would be prudent to do more than set the Editor right in matters of fact, and ask him to make the correction public without publishing your letter or mentioning your name? Otherwise, there are those who would say you were eager for notoriety. The road you tread of course lies through evil report as well as good, and when the evil comes you must "possess your soul in patience".'

Thus ended the best and most consecutive part of Elizabeth's training. She had spent a year in one of the principal teaching hospitals in London, she had received help and kindness and, no doubt, had acquired more insight into medical science and practice than the modern student in well-equipped laboratories in his first year. It was disappointing to leave the Middlesex, but her courage rose and she determined to get experience elsewhere and to qualify.

The next two months were spent at Aldeburgh and, while there, she heard from friends at the Middlesex Hospital and joined in family life.

E.G. to E.D.   *Aldeburgh, 10 Aug. 1861*
'I had a very kind letter from Mr. Heisch, the chemical lecturer, this morning, which I shall enclose for you

to read. It seems very pleasant to find a man not ashamed to rest a question at once on the most earnest ground, especially when I had not found him prone to talk religion. I have written him a long letter to-day, there is so much to say in answer to the yielding principle. To me the real question is, as I suppose it constantly is to every one, "What *is* God's will in this case?" '

E.G. to E.D.   *Aldeburgh, 11 Sept. 1861*

'I have just escaped from the family and a cricket match on the Grammar School lawn to write to you. We have had very little leisure as the house has been filled with visitors. We had thirteen besides our own family during last week, so you may imagine we were tolerably closely packed. I generally escape to an attic every morning after hearing the orders of the day, and read, write or do some chemistry in peace for an hour or two. My father is very restless about my plans, he cannot take in the fact that Greek and Mathematics with the sciences would be work enough for a winter, but talks despondently about not "feeling reconciled to my going back except I can enter a school". I really do not feel very anxious about entering a school this winter; the plan would be to be able to matriculate next summer at the London University or at St. Andrews, and begin the medical school work this time next year.'

One success occurred: Elizabeth received an undertaking [17 August 1861] from the Apothecaries' Hall.

Medical Training

She would be admitted to a qualifying examination for the licence when she had completed her studies 'according to the regulations of the court'. Her attention was called to a 'clause in our Act of Parliament which renders an apprenticeship of five years to a qualified medical practitioner imperative'. This arrangement had been discussed already with Mr. Plaskitt.

E.G. to E.D.   *Aldeburgh, 21 Aug. 1861*

'You will be almost as surprised and pleased as I am to hear that the Apothecaries are willing to examine me if I will go through the 5 years' apprenticeship and the usual routine of lectures, etc. Their decision reached me yesterday, and was welcomed with a "hurray" and congratulations all round the table. I have written to tell Mr. Plaskitt, and when my father is in London he must settle the apprenticeship question with him. We have rather a large party in the house and it does not seem friendly to absent oneself too much. We have been having picnics and other social sports lately and I have been grieved to find how unready I was with small talk and the gaiety that men desire in women. Knowing better things ought to raise oneself enough to make one capable of raising others or at least drawing their most interesting side out, though in reality it only seems able to make one slightly discontented with other people and yourself and longing for the higher kind of thing.'

The decision of the Society of Apothecaries assured

Medical Training

Elizabeth of a qualification, but she wanted a university degree as well as a licence. Could she gain admission at the University of London or at one of the Scottish universities? Her friend, Dr. Day (Professor of Anatomy and Medicine in the University of St. Andrews), was prepared to help her.

E.G. to E.D.   *3 Oct. 1861*
'I shall write a formal letter to St. Andrews this week to bring the question before the University Council there.'

Elizabeth noted: 'This winter can be spent very profitably in private work and for the matriculation at the London University or St. Andrews University.'

Refreshed and undismayed, Elizabeth returned to London where she attended some lectures on physiology by Professor Huxley.

E.G. to E.D.   *Manchester Sq., 19 Oct. 1861*
'We have been to Huxley's first lecture on Physiology this evening, and after it was over Miss Drewry, Miss Jex-Blake and the Misses Octavia and Miranda Hill came in and spent an hour with me. The lecture was very interesting and I felt sufficiently familiar with the subject matter to enjoy it very much. Miss Drewry dined here and went with me. She and the others have been having some metaphysical discussion on the origin of evil and individual responsibility. It is very pleasant to find

Medical Training

Maurice-like orthodoxy in Miss Jex-Blake's circle, it is
the want of something of this kind that prevents me
from completely enjoying the Drewrys, tho' they are
delightful morally and intellectually. I was introduced
to Huxley and he is now very kind in explaining and
pointing out different things. I wrote to Dr. Day about
10 days ago, reminding him of his promise to submit
my application to the Council as soon as the University
[St. Andrews] meets, and in answer, he sent the enclosed,
which you will not think very encouraging. He seemed
much more inclined to be a supporter, when he first
wrote two months ago, so I suppose he had been talking
to some disapproving old fogies.'

Character shows itself in adversity and during this
testing time, when rebuff and disappointment came
often, Elizabeth did not grow bitter or unhappy. Her
mouth may have become firmer, her lower lip more
prominent, but she remained serene and hopeful and,
while at Aldeburgh, she joined in the family life and
entertained visitors. Mr. Garrett doubted whether Elizabeth should leave Aldeburgh as her plans were uncertain. She thought differently. She must be at the centre
of affairs in London—able to consult her friends—and
she spent the autumn there with Louie. When in London, she helped every activity for the well-being of
women. 'The passion of my life is to help women,' is
a phrase in one of her letters. Miss Davies shared this

aspiration. No wonder these two should have meant so much to one another.

In 1859 Mme Bodichon had started an office in Langham Place to act as a bureau for helping women to find paid work. By 1861 Emily Davies, Elizabeth Garrett, Sophia Jex-Blake, Louie (Mrs. J. M. Smith), Emily Faithfull, Anne Proctor and many others met there. It was a centre of feminism and with hospital work in abeyance, Elizabeth had more time for this and other aspects of the women's movement. Jane Crowe became honorary secretary to the office. Youth, with burning aspiration and high ambition, thronged the little rooms. They were comrades and worked for a great end. The heart demands little beyond this. The need felt by women for openings to paid employment was written in the office books. Mrs. Smith said to her hairdresser: 'Surely, now, hairdressing is a calling suitable for women?' 'Impossible, madam,' he said, 'I myself took a fortnight to learn it.' Apart from medicine, Elizabeth found life full of interest: concerts, picture galleries, parties, sermons, especially those of the Rev. F. D. Maurice, who seemed a modern Isaiah after Mr. Dowler, all were grist to Elizabeth's mill. She was never ill and rarely tired. Elizabeth loved parties. She liked social intercourse, especially with 'superior people'. Miss Davies was not sure that it was justifiable to spend money on 'bonnets and flys', instead of instructive books. She wrote: 'Miss Garrett's case is different because successful physicians always consort with the aristocracy and she, of course, wishes to make her way in the world' (from a letter of Emily Davies quoted by Lady Stephen). Poor Elizabeth, a long road stretched between her and the goal of being a successful physician.

Elizabeth took the rebuff from the Middlesex well but this was only the beginning of the battle. At first her effort to study medicine was thought to be hardly worth serious notice, but as it became clear that she was in earnest and might storm her way into the fortress, then indeed its defenders paid her the compliment of prompt and strong opposition. It is not possible to trace in detail her experiences during the next four years but each medical school seems to have reacted much as the Middlesex Hospital did, its opposition being declared sooner and in more hostile terms. Her letters show that she kept her courage, her temper and even her sense of humour through a long series of exasperating trials. Again and again she was obliged to give up her training until a fresh opening could be found. During these intervals, when not with her parents, she stayed with Louie in London and joined in other efforts on behalf of women.

During the autumn of 1861 she was at Aldeburgh working at Greek and Latin. Her father grew restive— unless she had a definite plan, unless a medical school would accept her, it seemed to him a waste of time to learn a dead language! She approached teaching hospitals in London and they all refused her. Miss Davies and Elizabeth then turned their attention to the University of London which soon was to apply for a new charter: why not petition for a clause in it so that the degrees—arts and science as well as medicine—might be opened to women? Elizabeth asked to be allowed to matriculate and she began to prepare for the examination. A circular was sent to influential people inviting their support. Miss Davies took the lead in this effort and Elizabeth or her father paid the expense. Fifteen hundred leaflets were distributed and favourable replies were received among others from Mr. Gladstone, Mr. Cobden and Mrs. Mary Somerville. The petition to the University was nominally from Mr. Newson Garrett and it pointed out the immense advantage a university degree would be to governesses. Elizabeth wrote a full account of these efforts to Dr. Elizabeth Blackwell.

E.G. to E.B.   *22 Manchester Square, 8 May 1862*
'I have delayed writing; hoping that I might have good news of success to give you: now as this seems farther off than I had hoped it would be I will delay no longer. I think Mrs. Russell Gurney wrote you that I was spending all my time just now in preparing for the matriculation examination of the University of London. We made three very careful and vigorous efforts to gain admission of women into a medical school. Those we

tried were the Middlesex, the Westminster, and the London Hospitals; and early this year we attempted the Grosvenor Street School. I need not tell you we were in each case unsuccessful, though in one or two cases the adverse decision was gained by a very small majority of votes. In each case those gentlemen who opposed always urged as one ground for their doing so, that as the examining bodies were not prepared to admit women to their examinations the school could not educate a woman to be an illegal practitioner, and that by doing so they would incur the certain risk of injuring the school in the eyes of the public without really aiding women. The medical papers also took up the same line. The *Lancet* was particularly anxious to point out that we were beginning at the wrong end, and that the first thing we should do was to settle the question of examinations. I therefore applied to the Apothecaries' Hall and to the College of Surgeons asking the latter body if they would allow me to compete for the special diploma in midwifery which they now give. This was refused. The application to the [Apothecaries'] Hall was more fortunate: the question turned on a legal technicality and was referred to counsel and finally decided in my favour. I must, of course, conform to all the ordinary regulations but when I have done so I can obtain the licence to practise granted by that body. One of the regulations I have met without difficulty—viz. being apprenticed to a medical man for five years before the final examination. I had indentures made out as soon as I knew the decision. The second one (spending three years in a medical school in the United Kingdom) is more difficult. Still as the licence is not all I want I thought it better to make an effort at some university for the M.D. For many reasons it seems desirable to make the attempt at the London University. It was clear that the only chance of obtaining admission to the examinations lay in keeping the question on the widest, most general ground, advocating the claims of governesses and other women who required a good general examination, without introducing the question of medical degrees or the admission of woman to any new professions. The University is about to have a new Charter and we therefore thought that this was the time to raise the question by praying the Senate to obtain the insertion of a clause expressly extending to women the benefits of their examinations. Before doing this we had submitted the present charter to the Attorney-General and had had his opinion upon the power of the Senate to admit women upon its authority as it is now drawn up. He thought they had no power to do so and therefore there was no alternative but to ask for a new clause.

'In order to get some expression of the general feeling on the question circulars were extensively distributed and as a result we obtained a very respectable number of names as allies. The Vice-Chancellor and Mrs. Grote were throughout most kindly ready to help us and to give the proposal the full weight of their influence. The discussion at the Senate came on yesterday and was a most lengthened and animated one; of twenty-one members present, ten were for, ten against and one neutral. The Chancellor [Lord Granville] then had the casting vote and gave it against us. I am exceedingly sorry, as this would have been fraught with such great benefit to many different classes of women. However this is not to be had now; perhaps when they are having another charter eight or ten years hence, we may try again and succeed. I do not imagine there is much chance of being able to do more at any other university in the United Kingdom than we can do here so that I fear the possibility of ever obtaining an English degree as M.D. is a very remote one.

'My notion now is to try to get into a school and obtain the Apothecaries' Hall licence. If this should prove possible it would occupy between three and four years from next October. My own feeling is in favour of having the M.D., though it should be a foreign one I believe it would command more respect than the licence from the Hall would alone.'

After being refused by the University of London, and also by the Universities of Oxford and Cambridge, it was decided that application to any other English university would be useless. The Scottish universities were considered next.

Medical Training

Mr. Newson Garrett consulted Mr. Justice Hannen about the possibility of either St. Andrews or Glasgow University allowing a woman to take their medical examinations.

Mr. Justice Hannen to Newson Garrett
London, 26 Nov. 1862

'I have not seen the charter of St. Andrews or Glasgow, I am therefore unable to form an opinion on the legal questions: (1) whether either University has the power to admit a woman to matriculation; (2) whether a woman has a right to be so admitted. I think it improbable that there is any University where a woman has a right to be admitted, but if it can be established that any University in the United Kingdom has the power to admit, a great step will have been made towards ultimate success. I was obliged to come to the conclusion that the University of London has not the power—I suppose that the Lord Advocate has expressed a similar opinion with regard to St. Andrews. On the other hand I came to the conclusion, in an analogous case, that the Society of Apothecaries had the power to admit a woman to examination. . . .'

In November 1862 Elizabeth went to Scotland, having first assured herself that attendance at lectures in a Scottish university would be accepted by the authorities of the Apothecaries' Hall.

Elizabeth went to St. Andrews first in the hope of

gaining admission to lectures there and, if possible, permission to matriculate as the preliminary step to a degree. If she failed there, she would go to Edinburgh. She had friends at both places.

She wrote to her sister, Louie, on the way to St. Andrews after a few days in Edinburgh that, 'The ferry across the Firth of Forth was primitive, the loss of luggage overboard being a common catastrophe.'

Dr. Day, Regius Professor of Medicine, was friendly and helpful but, unfortunately, he could not attend meetings unless they were held in his house. He was not above helping with advice, however, as to the taking of the University fort by surprise.

E.G. to L.M.S. St. Andrews (*undated*), *Nov. 1862*

'About 11 Miss Otté [probably secretary to Dr. Day] came in. She came rather primed with difficulties; the professors were so afraid for me; the students are so particularly rough here, and will certainly insult me; Dr. Heddle's chemical class is absolutely essential to make up the first medical year and he is a timid man just new to office who would particularly object to doing anything singular; also it was essential that I should matriculate before getting tickets for any class, and as soon as I presented myself for that the question would be referred to the whole Senatus who would probably refuse to sanction anything so novel. Finally Miss Otté herself thought the scheme impracticable. I was rather relieved to hear this, as I thought it might have tinged all the rest to a certain extent; however, she was very kind and ended by asking me to go for a walk round the town with her to end with a call upon Dr. Day. It was a lovely winter's day, keen and bright, with the very clear grey-blue sky one only sees in cold weather. . . . About 12½ we went in to Dr. Day; he spoke again about the matriculation and advised I should try for it as soon as possible. I thought of course it was an examination but to my joy he said, "No, it is merely a fee of £1, for which a student receives a ticket as a member of the University and upon the strength of which he is allowed to take tickets for the several classes." The man who gives these tickets has the character of being very wide-awake and certain never to put his head into a snoose [*sic*] so that the chances were he would say he must consult the Senatus when he heard my request. Miss Otté and I sallied out at once to him, and I stated that I was going to attend Dr. Day's class and that he had informed me I must first receive a matriculation ticket. I was careful only to mention Dr. Day's one class, which is very small and which he might fancy I was attending for some whim. To my delight the dear old buffer quietly said "Oh, very weel," and pulled down the University ledger, told me to write my name, which I did gleefully, received the coin (such small change I thought it was for that precious card) and gave me instead a card bearing the desired magic words:

Medical Training

"Civis Universitatis Andrewesis" beneath my name, which being translated recognize me as a member of this ancient and august, etc. etc. I don't know what lever the Senatus might find available for returning me the £1 (declined with thanks) but I suspect they have put themselves *hors de combat* by this deed. They may protest, but surely a name once on their books has a good chance of remaining there. Any one professor may refuse to admit me into his classroom, but I shall be moderate and not ask for any I can do without. Dr. Day's and Dr. Heddle's I *must* have, and getting them it will be my aim to keep very quiet and in the background so that the wrath of the enemy be not needlessly roused. Dr. Day was greatly elated with the success, and sent us off to Dr. Heddle to secure his ticket before the opponents know what is done. Dr. H. has promised well to Dr. Day and wishes to please him, so I have good hope all will be well. I sent a letter home to-day with the bare fact of the matriculation business being well over, as I only came home just in time for the mid-day post. Perhaps if you are writing you could send dear Mother this fuller account. I shall write to her after seeing Dr. H.'

E.G. to L.M.S.　　　　　　　*St. Andrews, Nov. 1862*

'I have been writing so much to dear Father that you will feel quite up to all my news of the last few days though I have not written to you. I cannot tell you how

Medical Training

much pleasure dear Father's kind letters have given me, it is wonderfully good of him not to get tired of these continual struggles and fights. Not having any interest in the subjects in the meantime, must make the unpleasant parts seem the only prominent thing in the business. The Senatus resolved to-day to send back the matriculation fee, so when I returned from walking with Mrs. Day this afternoon, I found Mr. MacBean (the poor man who gave me the ticket) waiting for me. He seemed very uncomfortable and at last said he *never* had had anything to do which he hated so much, indeed he did not deserve my kindness and that's it! and at the word he deposited a little paper wrappage on the table. I looked mystified and he added: "Oh! ma'am, it's the fee! I can't help it, etc. etc." So I asked him to be comforted as to his share, I knew he had no more to do with it than I had, but that he must pick it up again for receive it I would not. He said the orders of the Senatus were positive and that he must leave it, so I said I should return it in an envelope as soon as he left the house, which I have done, adding a letter to say that till the question was decided legally against my being allowed to retain the matriculation ticket, I could not consent to have the fee paid for the same returned to me. So he will have to inform the Senatus that this will not answer. Father's telegram came while Mr. MacBean was here so I got the information for my answer straight from him. Dr. Tulloch [Principal and Primarius Pro-

Medical Training

fessor of St. Mary's College, the theological side of the University] came to Dr. Day before the meeting to-day, and Dr. Day took the opportunity to use his powers of persuasion on my behalf. When reported, they were to the effect that my father had this matter very much at heart, and would be glad to employ some *very* able person to investigate the whole question connected with the ancient right of women to graduate, and would not think 100 guineas too much to give for such investigation provided it was found possible to admit me. Dr. Day had thought of doing it himself, but it had occurred to him that it was more in Tulloch's way than his! So off went the Vice-Chancellor to the meeting chewing the cud of reflection over this hint, and when he came back afterwards, by his own account he had been standing up for me very gallantly! The Senatus are acting with some want of generosity in refusing to hold any of their meetings in Dr. Day's house. They often do so in ordinary cases, and just now he is suffering so much from his knee that he could not attempt to get even as far as he does occasionally. However the special committee appointed to consider the question will meet in his room to-morrow. One of his old pupils still a student of the University came to see him to-day, and Dr. Day asked what the feeling was among the students, and he said they were almost to a man on my side, so much so that when some allusion was made in the introductory lecture to-day to the advances of female education by my arch-enemy,

Medical Training

Forbes [Principal Forbes, the theologian], there was a regular tumult of cries of applause, they taking the opportunity of showing their sentiments. Their feeling is that the Senatus is treating me very unjustly. This student told Dr. Day that the senior students of the two colleges [the United College of St. Salvator and St. Leonard, secular, and St. Mary's College, theological] were to meet to-night and consider the question and if (as he thinks certain) they pass a resolution unanimously approving of my admission, a general meeting of all the students will be called, and a memorial prepared for their signature expressive of their good feeling in the matter. Even if we fail ultimately, to have all the 3 medical professors [Professors Day, Heddle and Wm. Macdonald] and the students on my side, will be good points.'

There seemed to be danger of a lawsuit between Elizabeth and the University. Neither side wanted this. As it was, the affair attracted publicity and there was an article about it in the *Spectator* which Elizabeth feared might antagonize the Senatus still more.

E.G. to L.M.S.   *St. Andrews (undated)*
'Nothing has happened since I wrote, but I think the general irritation is subsiding, and the Senatus is growing daily less inclined to rush into a lawsuit, so I am in hopes the threat of one will do instead, I should horribly dislike swamping a lot of money in law, in fact when it came

Medical Training

to the last I don't think in justice to the other children that we could really risk going into a suit, unless it were made a public question, the expenses to be defrayed by subscription. However the folk here have a magnificent idea of our wealth, and it is all right for them to think we could rush upon them in law without an instant's hesitation on our own account. Please *do* send my studs and miscroscope key. I think they would come safely in cotton wool, in the farther corner (from the stamp) of a large envelope. We are going to dine with some enemies to-night—the Sellars[1]—I hope to meet some more enemies. I shall wear my light silk and appear as rich as I can! This is such an education for low cunning. I only wish your rings were within reach! Had we rightly considered the matter, perhaps you would have lent them to me during the storm, to help me to overcome the Senatus.'

E.G. to L.M.S.　　　　　　　*St. Andrews, December*

'Thanks for the studs and key—they came yesterday and I have been studying the tongue of a limpet, and the suckers of an echinus all the morning with the microscope, and enjoying unpacking it very much. It was quite uninjured. I dare say you have heard from some of the home party about Sir F. Kelly's [Solicitor-General and Attorney-General] opinion. It was sadly against us.

[1] William Young Sellar, Professor of Humanity [Latin] at St. Andrews University.

Medical Training

He said decidedly that the Senatus *could* not admit a woman, even if they wished to do so, as the Charter stands now, such a thing would be impossible. This was of course very unpleasant, but I stuck the letter into my deepest petticoat pocket and determined to say nothing to any one here about it, not even to my friends, thinking that while the knowledge of its contents was confined to me and my petticoat pocket, they would not do so much harm as they were capable of doing if they came to the enemies' ears. I had hard work not to tell Dr. Day and Miss Otté, especially as they knew I was expecting to hear from Sir F. Kelly, but I did manage not to give even a hint of having had any communication with him.

'Yesterday Mr. Campbell Smith [advocate in Edinburgh] had a consultation with the Lord Advocate of Scotland,[1] and to my joy he entirely differs from Sir F. Kelly, being quite clear that the charter does *not* make it impossible for a woman to attend college classes, though he admits that a considerable discretionary power rests with the Senatus, they may, in his opinion, refuse any one, male or female, if they think it necessary to do so. I am greatly delighted with his view. Of course the Senatus may now stand out on their own responsibility, but they know that in doing so they lay themselves open to an action. I believe that by granting me tickets, they have thrown away their discretionary power, as far as I

[1] James Moncrieff, Lord Advocate for Scotland, 1864.

am concerned. They meet to-day to consider the matter. Dr. Day cannot get up some horrid steps leading to their Council room, so that he cannot be there either.'

Miss Emily Davies joined Elizabeth at St. Andrews during the struggle. It was a sign of great friendship to take the long, uncomfortable, expensive journey in the winter. No doubt her presence solaced Elizabeth much and helped her to face the difficulties. In the end, the University refused to allow her to take the general course of lectures, but she remained for the winter session working privately under Professor Day.

Mrs. Russell Gurney in a letter of sympathy seemed to assume that the fight was over.

Mrs. R.G. to E.G.   *London, 1 Dec. 1862*

'I do hope you have not for a moment thought we were unmindful of you in this most disappointing affair, though I have been silent. Now I have very much come to the conclusion that after all it does not so very much matter because if the time is not come for women to enter the profession—one woman would not hasten much its coming, by entering as an exceptional case and I know you think more of the *cause* than of your *personal* success. Perhaps you help on the cause most by being what you are, and perhaps you grow best in being, by not ranking amongst the successful: this is how I comfort myself.'

During the following summer (1863) Elizabeth spent

Medical Training

some months in Edinburgh, working under Professor
Simpson and Dr. Keiller, but the University refused her
as a student and she had to withdraw. With this rebuff
she broke down; it was monotonously disappointing:
so many blows and no success. But courage and hope
returned speedily. She wrote that she had recovered her
spirits with 'my usual speed'.

Later in the year she was in London again, staying
with Louie. Her plan was to pass the Apothecaries' Hall
examination and then to supplement its licence by a
foreign medical degree. The pressing need was experience in dissection and she wrote to various medical men
asking for instruction and offering a high fee for it.

A letter to Dr. Canton of Charing Cross may be
quoted as a sample of many similar ones.

E.G. to Dr. C.C.   *London, 25 July 1863*
'I am anxious to obtain such a course of instruction in
anatomy as shall enable me to pass the examination of
the Apothecaries' Hall. As I am aware of the difficulties
in the way of my being allowed to have lectures given
to other students, I wrote some few months ago to the
Court of Examiners, asking if they would accept a certificate of private lectures if given by a recognized
teacher and if equal to the course usually given in public.
As a result of the enquiry the following resolution was
passed in the next meeting of the Court. Resolved:
"That Miss Garrett be informed that the Court of

Medical Training

Examiners only demand that the certificates on the various subjects required by the Court be obtained from recognized Lecturers of acknowledged schools of medicine." I should be glad to offer a fee of 25 guineas for the anatomy certificate required by the Hall or to make any other arrangement the Lecturer may prefer.'

From Aldeburgh where she was paying a visit, she wrote to Miss Davies, 'I enjoy coming back very much but I would not return permanently for anything.'

'I want surgical knowledge constantly,' she wrote and, 'must study it now as best I may'. She wrote to more medical men, in the attempt to get teaching in dissection and surgical anatomy. One was as far away as Aberdeen and his reply shows that some of the answers she received were not pleasant.

Mr. I.H. to E.G.   *Aberdeen, 29 July 1863*
'I must decline to give you instruction in Anatomy. My time is so occupied in other things as to leave me no leisure for private tuition—but, apart from this, I have so strong a conviction that the entrance of ladies into dissecting-rooms and anatomical theatres is undesirable in every respect, and highly unbecoming that I could not do anything to promote your end. Your money would only be thrown away in fees for lectures, unless you would wish to seek, and could find some anatomical lecturer prepared to give you admission with the other students into the dissecting-room. I leave you to judge

whether that would be desirable. It is indeed necessary for the purpose of Surgery and Medicine that these matters should be studied, but fortunately it is not necessary that fair ladies should be brought into contact with such foul scenes—nor would it be for their good any more than for that of their patients if they could succeed in leaving the many spheres of usefulness which God has pointed out to them in order to force themselves into competition with the lower walks of the medical profession. Ladies would make bad doctors at the best, and they do so many things excellently that I for one should be sorry to see them trying to do this one. I should be extremely glad to hear that further reflexion had led you to be of my opinion.'

Another wrote saying: 'Believe me I am among the warmest advocates for the cultivation of the mind of woman but I will never consent to unsex them.' Each letter was a slap in the face and they came continually. She must have dreaded the postman's knock.

In the midst of these discouragements we find Elizabeth writing:

E.G. to E.D.   *London, 3 Nov. 1863*
'Did you feel All Saints' Day to be encouraging? It sounds horribly conceited but I did, very. Every one who is yearning and struggling for liberty and larger light—for the coming of the Lord—*must* take heart as he looks at all those whom he succeeds.'

Medical Training

After repeated disappointments, permission was obtained, in February 1864, for Elizabeth to visit the wards of the London Hospital, again in the nominal capacity of a nurse but with leisure for study. She also obtained instruction in anatomy from the professor and demonstrator of anatomy in the medical school. She lived in lodgings in Philpot Street, a turning off the Commercial Road, and attended midwifery cases in the district.

E.G. to E.D. *Philpot St., 3 Feb. 1864*

'I feel seedy this morning from not having been to bed, two cases filled up every moment from 6 last night to 10 this morning. The last was exceedingly interesting as being my first case of operative midwifery. When I found the difficulty I made up my mind what I should like to do but thought it wiser to call in Mr. Heckford. When he came he agreed to my plan of treatment and kindly left me everything to do except giving the chloroform. It was not a minor operation and I enjoyed it immensely.'

E.G. to E.D. *Philpot St., 16 Feb. 1864*

'I went down to Vere St. in time for the morning sermon (too late for anything else!). It was fine to stand in the gallery and see the dear old prophet [Rev. F. D. Maurice] with the knowledge of what he felt about the two things I was full of. His letter in the *Spectator* is grand.

'I have been to the London Hospital this morning for

Medical Training

the first time and am now going again. It is distressingly
nervous work, standing about with nothing definite to
do and the consciousness of being under a fire of criticizing eyes, nurses', patients' and students'. But this stage
does not last long, when the novelty goes off they look
less and you feel less, thank goodness. I live here still and
shall do as they have no room to give me.'

E.G. to E.D.   Philpot St., 18 Feb. 1864
'Thanks for your letter. I agree with you in thinking
snubbing won't be a serious evil in the long run, still it
is unpleasant and for a time hindering. You cannot at
once believe that personal effort can altogether make up
for all the help that teaching and guidance give other
students. To-day after I had been round a few beds with
Dr. Powell he took me into the nurses' room and told
me he had been officially ordered not to allow me to go
round the wards with him, and that as he was only a
subaltern he was reluctantly obliged to obey. So I must
peg away alone and do as well as I can. It is harder work
and far less interesting—besides the painful sense of conflict which I must have whenever an enemy comes into
the ward—but still the self-reliant frame it puts me into
will be good, it will force me to look closer than I would
be likely to do if I had any one to appeal to in every
difficulty. Mr. Heckford reports that some of the elder
students are warmly on my side, so that perhaps in time
I may find them out and be able to ask them questions

III

in cases of puzzlement, and as a last resort I shall get Mr. Heckford to come and help me. He says the storm is going down but that he never saw the school in such an uproar about anything before. They seem to have dwelt particularly on the shabbiness of my pretending to be a nurse, but as I said that was not my fault, I had given them two chances of having me as a regular student.'

The atmosphere of disapproval weighed on her more at the London Hospital than it had done three years earlier at the Middlesex. The conflict had been going on a long time and perhaps also the burden of hostility was not lightened by friendships such as she had found before.

Miss Davies tried to enlist help from influential laymen.

E.G. to E.D.   *Philpot St., 10 April 1864*
'Thank you very much for going to the Grotes. It was a courageous piece of help to give. I am not at all sanguine about the decision at the London Hospital. The instinct with all bodies is so conservative and they may plainly see that the obstructive interest will be best served by woman practitioners being as unfit really as it is said they will be. I have had a skirmish with the arch-enemy here, Dr. P., which has ended in a kind of drawn result. I yield the point about going round the wards with him and he yields, I believe, the greater part of his personal animosity. He will not again order the resident medical

officer to cut me. I told him my mind about that and I think he was ashamed. The battle took place at his house this morning. I had heard of his saying nasty things and I determined to stop it if possible. It was a horrid errand but my courage rose at the right moment and I was able to express myself calmly as well as strongly. We had never spoken before; he became wonderfully civil and pleasant before we finished, the talk lasted more than ½ hour.'

It is not known exactly what happened at the London Hospital to bring about her expulsion after working there for six months.

In October 1864 she left the London Hospital and was again with Louie, in Manchester Square. Another period of solitary work followed. Perhaps Mr. Joshua Plaskitt's help belongs to this period as well as to many of the other intervals of hospital training. Prompted by friends on the staff of the Middlesex Hospital, Elizabeth asked permission to visit the wards without recognition as a student. 'I request only permission to enter the wards as a visitor.' In reply she was told that it was not within the province of the medical committee to grant a general permission, but that each physician and surgeon had power to grant permission at his discretion for his own wards or ward. Thus Elizabeth returned to the Middlesex Hospital and persevered under these rather unsatisfactory terms during the following five months.

Medical Training

At the end of March 1865 this arrangement also ended, by decision of the medical committee. The various doctors who had allowed her access to their wards wrote rescinding their permission, some quite kindly. Elizabeth's connection with the Middlesex Hospital was at an end. In spite of disappointments, her debt to the hospital and to the medical staff was great and, on the whole, she had happy memories of the Middlesex. She had made many friends amongst the staff and the training she received there was invaluable.

Perhaps repeated disappointments made Elizabeth a little off-handed with Miss Davies, who wrote to reprove her in two extremely earnest letters.

E.D. to E.G.   *1 July 1865*
'My complaint is that from the very beginning you have assumed that you *knew*, and did not want advice or help from anybody. I don't think it is the reiteration of advice that made you turn away from it. I did not want you to come to *me* for advice, tho' I might have been able to give some hints, and I did not want you to bind yourself down to take anybody's advice. That is a different thing from listening to it respectfully. I think perhaps your way of receiving a suggestion (*advice* is too large and strong a word) by contradiction, leaves one with the impression that you have not exactly heard it with your mental ear, and are not going to entertain it, and that may lead to provoking reiteration. The slightest

intimation that you intended to consider it, would of course make repetition unnecessary. Things of no consequence one does not press, but if it seems to me an important matter, I am tempted to go on, in a way which is no doubt worrying I should like very much to know whether it is only the thing, or partly my manner of doing it, that is provoking. Of course one has no right to do it at all, unless it is wished, and if you tell me that you would rather be let alone, I shall offer no more advice. I should be sorry, because, tho' I don't think you are dependent upon advice to keep you straight, it seems to me that in a position so peculiarly difficult and ensnaring as yours is likely to be, the hints of a bystander might often save you from making mistakes, and except Louie, there is no one who will ever tell you anything. But what I want to know is whether, *when* I see things, you would like best for me to speak or to keep silence. I cannot go on speaking freely, if there is any kind of impression on your side that I do it to relieve myself, not distinctly in obedience to your own desire.

'Whichever way you decide, I should like you to go on criticizing me, a great deal more freely than you do. I believe I don't mind being told things half as much as most people.'

E.D. to E.G.   *3 July 1865*
'I am glad to find that my letter does not seem to have hurt you quite so much as I was afraid it might. But I

don't think we quite understand each other yet. I never thought that you despised advice, *when* you "acknowledge the fitness of the giver and feel in need of advice". My regret is that you so seldom do either, and especially the last. As to the giver, of course the matter is very complicated and can scarcely be judged of generally. I am surprised that you prefer criticism of things *done*. I carefully refrain from it, on the principle that it would be giving useless pain. I am sure also that the same temper of mind which resents criticism of *proposed* plans, would be equally offended by criticism afterwards. That is, it would refuse to acknowledge failure. As far as I can see, there is no one, except Louie and myself, with whom you are in the habit of discussing plans on quite free and equal terms (if you are with us?). There is no one I believe, who would venture to offer a suggestion without being expressly asked and you don't ask. In this you differ from other people. It is rather curious that we should in a manner have changed places in this matter. One would have thought that I should be more sensitive than you. Perhaps the reason may be that I am so keenly alive to the unspoken criticism (sometimes expressed by unconscious look or manner) and give it credit for such extreme severity, that anything said is mildness itself by comparison. You probably take for granted that people are liking and approving when nothing is said to the contrary, while I am apt to take the opposite for granted. No doubt the difference in our family atmospheres tells.

Medical Training

Yours is one of mutual admiration, rather conspicuously
manifested. Mine is the reverse, at least the negative.
And that, added on to natural temperament, is very
likely to make you confident and me doubtful. We
ought both to take care not to let our respective peculiarities go too far.'

Miss Davies' letters on this occasion have been kept
and Elizabeth's destroyed.

For years Emily Davies had looked upon Elizabeth as
her 'public work'. Perhaps the fact that her protégée was
growing up prompted her to turn to other aspects of the
movement. At any rate, by this time Miss Davies was
spending much thought on the admission of women in
general to the Higher Local University Examinations and
to starting Hitchin College.

In the autumn of 1865 Elizabeth's struggle was end-
ing. By adding one course of lectures to another, and by
the invaluable help of Mr. Plaskitt, after spending nearly
six years in constant study and having passed with credit
all her preliminary examinations, she had completed the
curriculum imposed on candidates for a medical diploma.
She was able to apply to the Society of Apothecaries—
the only examining body that was unable by the terms
of its charter to exclude her as a woman. The board of
examiners, forgetful of their undertaking four years previously, wished to refuse. However, Mr. Garrett issued
an ultimatum and threatened legal action, with the result

that she sat for the examination, passing with credit, and obtained the diploma, L.S.A. A year later her name appeared in the Medical Register.

In order to prevent other women taking the L.S.A., the Society of Apothecaries altered its regulations. In the future candidates for their diploma must have worked in a recognized medical school, and from these women were excluded.

As soon as Elizabeth qualified, Mr. Garrett leased a house for her, No. 20 Upper Berkeley Street. He also gave her furniture and pictures. What should Elizabeth put on her door plate? Every detail is important to a pioneer. She wrote, 'I don't like "Miss Garrett" on the door. It is only like a dressmaker. Louie strongly advises for "Elizabeth Garrett, L.S.A." and a night bell.'

However engrossing her profession was, Elizabeth made time for general reading.

E.G. to E.D.   *Aldeburgh, 12 Sept. 1865*
'Thanks for your long letter this morning. I must read Milton on *Divorce*, it must be fine to see him taking the noble line of argument in such a question. Arnold's life, with all the pathetic craving for sympathy which strikes you so much, is very familiar to me. I never read any book with the same degree of sympathy which it called out when I was in the chrysalis stage after leaving school. It came as a real gospel to me to find any one at once as liberal and as Christian as Arnold was. I suppose to every

one, in the state I was then in, light in some measure
comes sooner or later, and that if Arnold had not come
in my way something else would have done the same
for me, but still one remembers the light-bearer with
unusual reverence. Arnold's life is not a mere book to
me but a sort of Bible which came when it was wanted.'

5

THE PARIS M.D.

>>❯❯❯●❮❮❮<<

When Elizabeth Garrett passed the milestone of qualification, the worst of her struggle was over and the
character of her life changed. She started the St. Mary's
Dispensary which became the New Hospital for Women, and of which an account will be given later. She
made a success of general practice and yet found time
for public work, for concerts, picture galleries and
society. Friends who had sympathized with her difficulties consulted her, for to go to a medical woman was
the proof of their belief in women doctors.

In 1865 women did not possess the parliamentary
franchise in any country in the world. In that year,
however, John Stuart Mill, standing as parliamentary
candidate for Westminster, focused attention upon the
question. Although his views were unusual, the constituency was eager to secure him as its representative.
He refused to canvass or to spend money on the contest,
on the ground that it was a public service to sit in
Parliament and that money spent by the candidate on
the election amounted to buying the seat. Worse fol-

lowed; in his election address he stated that, if returned, he meant to do his utmost to secure for women the parliamentary franchise on the same terms as it was or might be granted to men. A reform bill was imminent and Mme Bodichon called upon him to offer her help and to ask what could be done to press the claims of women. Mill agreed to present a petition from women householders if he were returned to Parliament. As election day approached, Mme. Bodichon and Miss Davies toured the constituency in an open carriage, no doubt displaying appropriate colours and posters. 'Giving our support to Mr. Mill,' the former called it, but as the voters said, 'Mr. Mill wants girls in Parliament,' it is doubtful if they helped him much. In spite of Mill's views he was successful, and sat at Westminster for the three sessions which passed the Reform Bill, 1867. To the women he said: 'Give me something I can brandish with effect'; thereupon the office in Langham Place hummed with activity and Miss Garrett, at last a householder, offered rooms for additional work. 'I have a distinct recollection', wrote Miss Emily Davies in the *Family Chronicle*, 'of the party of friends who met at Miss Garrett's house from day to day and worked at it [the petition]. One of the early signatures that we hailed with special delight was that of Mrs. Alford, the name and the address—the Deanery, Canterbury—being so highly respectable!'[1]

[1] Reprinted from *Emily Davies and Girton College* by Barbara Stephen.

The Paris M.D.

It was about this time that Professor Huxley published his support of the enfranchisement of women. He wrote: 'The fact is we are still in the harem stage, though in the last stage of it, and those men who like to keep women in the doll stage are not out of it.' On 7 June 1866 the petition with 1,500 signatures was taken to the House of Commons. It was in the name of Barbara L. Bodichon and others, but some of the active promoters could not come and the honour of presenting it fell to Emily Davies and Elizabeth Garrett. Miss Garrett liked to be ahead of time, so the delegation arrived early in the Great Hall, Westminster, she with the roll of parchment in her arms. It made a large parcel and she felt conspicuous. To avoid attracting attention she turned to the only woman who seemed, among the hurrying men, to be a permanent resident in that great shrine of memories, the apple-woman, who agreed to hide the precious scroll under her stand; but, learning what it was, insisted first on adding her signature, so the parcel had to be unrolled again. Mill proposed the amendment to the Reform Bill in May of the following year, an account of his speech being found in Lady Amberley's diary.[1] 'Disraeli first made a short statement . . . at ¼ to 8 Mill got up at once to move his first amendment on clause 4 that the word person should be inserted instead of the word man. The house was very thin but he was listened to with the utmost attention and respect. He came to a most painful

[1] *Amberley Papers* ed. by Bertrand & Patricia Russell.

pause at one time nr. the beginning of his speech and stood silent for near 2 minutes or more; he seemed quite lost, only his eyebrows worked fearfully; the House cheered him and he resumed and went on fluently to the end. .... Denham spoke for Mill and Fawcett[1] and 2 others against him, all those against him were silly and frivolous and without argument. The division was at 10 o'clock and the numbers were with Mr. Mill 73 against 196. .... Mill was much pleased and every one was surprised at the number for him.'

In the opinion of Mill himself, his action in bringing about the first parliamentary debate on women's suffrage was by far the most important service he rendered in the House of Commons. In his autobiography Mill recorded: 'For women not to make their claim to the suffrage at the time when the elective franchise was being largely extended would have been to abjure the claim altogether and a movement on the subject was begun in 1866 when I presented a petition for the suffrage signed by a considerable number of distinguished women. But it was as yet uncertain whether the proposal would obtain more than a few stray votes in the House and when after a Debate in which the speakers on the opposite side were conspicuous by their feebleness, the vote recorded in favour of the motion amounted to 73, the surprise was general and the encouragement great.'

[1] This sentence is slightly ambiguous but of course Fawcett supported Mill.

The Paris M.D.

The campaign thus launched continued until success came in 1918 and in the following year Miss Emily Davies, eighty-nine years of age, walked to the poll.

There are several references to Miss Garrett in Lady Amberley's diary. They shared the same hopes for women and the understanding of the younger woman for the needs of less well-placed women made her a valuable ally. She and Elizabeth became friends. She went to a lecture on physiology given by Miss Garrett in March 1866. 'Every one cared for it more than I did,' she wrote. Shortly afterwards she and Lord Amberley visited J. S. Mill at Blackheath, where his step daughter, Miss Helen Taylor, received them. Lady Amberley's diary records: 'later came Mr. Herbert Spencer (the philosopher) and Mr. Hill, an editor of the *Daily News* and Miss Garrett the woman doctor whom I had heard lecture on Physiology at her own house. She and I had been asked on purpose to meet one another, as I wanted to know her. We dined at 6 (excellent dinner) delightful general talk, it was most pleasant. The talk was on Comte, G. Evans (G. Eliot) and her new book *Felix Holt* . . . on H. Spencer's theory of the sun coming to an end and losing all its force. . . . At 10 they sent us and Miss Garrett home together in their carriage and we had a nice talk on the way home. Her dispensary opens next week. She had much difficulty in becoming a doctor fr. want of facility for women to learn. She wd. not mind attending men but does not do it, on account of what wd. be said. We got home at 11 having enjoyed our day immensely.'

In 1867 Elizabeth faced the chief sorrow of her life. Her sister Louie, Mrs. J. W. Smith, died from appendicitis after a short illness, leaving four young children. Louie had been a perfect elder sister. Her grace and beauty were combined with ability and character. She was one of the few people to whom Elizabeth turned for advice. They had been inseparable, and even after Louie's marriage Elizabeth had lived with her almost continuously. 'Our darling is gone and we can never get a word or look from her again!' It is the cry that has arisen from broken hearts through the ages: the cry of the one who is left for the one who has gone. It touches the mystery that cannot be solved. In her practical way, Elizabeth felt that to care for Louie's children was the way to show her love for Louie, as, indeed, she had promised while Louie lay dying. 'Don't be unhappy about the children,' she said. 'Your children shall be as mine even if I have my own,' and she wrote to her sister Alice, married and in India, 'I have now a feeling against ever marrying in order to keep my best love and keenest interests for them' [Louie's children]. Every few days, whatever her engagements, Elizabeth went to see them. 'My children,' she called them. Outings, treats, and discipline when required were much considered by her during the coming years. The boys went to school and passed from her; on the girls she lavished love and care. Louie's influence with her family did not die with her.

The Paris M.D.

Years later what her opinion would have been was a matter of interest still. Mrs. Garrett writing to Elizabeth in 1897 said: 'Our dear Louie must have been a lovely strong character to be so present with us all as she is now after 30 years of visible absence from us.'

A letter of sympathy in this great sorrow came from Miss Sophia Jex-Blake, who was then in America, in contact with women physicians, whose work inspired her later to adopt medicine as her career.

Miss S.J.-B. to E.G.   *10 April 1867*
'I think you know how much I cared for your sister and how highly I prized her friendship. I do not think that I can tell you how deeply grieved I am at her loss for my own sake, and yet how I feel that my sorrow can be nothing to yours. Perhaps you and I have not always understood each other so well as she and I did, but I want you to know how heartily and painfully I sympathize with you, and how I wish that I could take your hand and tell you so. One thought that has been very present in my mind since first the rumour reached me is of all the talks and wonderings we have had together, you and she and I, and how now perhaps it is all plain and clear to her—"Now she knows what Rhamses knows"—while we are left to moil and puzzle on through this terrible tangle of things which used to perplex us all alike. I think I need hardly tell you how glad I should be to hear from you anything that you like

to tell me, and yet that I shall not at all expect or wish you to write to me unless you feel like it.'

An effort was made in 1866 to introduce continental methods into England for the control of venereal disease and in that year the first of the Contagious Diseases Acts was passed. The principle of state regulation and compulsory examination of prostitutes had been practised in France and some other European countries since the time of Napoleon and statistics were quoted to prove that these methods controlled the spread of the disease. The prevalence of venereal disease in England was serious and the medical profession strongly supported parliamentary action. The regulations at first affected garrison towns only, but other acts followed, widening the sphere of action. Immediate and vigorous opposition arose. In the constituencies, this was led by Mrs. Josephine Butler, a woman of saintly life and intense courage; while in the House of Commons the protagonist for abolition was the Rt. Hon. Sir James Stansfeld, who sacrificed his political career and spent twenty years working for the repeal of the Acts. Mrs. Butler and her supporters were convinced that the group of feminist women would support abolition. Dr. Elizabeth Blackwell did so. Miss Garrett did not. She accepted the prevalent view of the profession that, distasteful as the measures were, they provided the only means of protecting innocent people—mainly women and children—from venereal disease. She has been severely criticized for supporting the regulations. During the controversy, which was most bitter, she wrote to the press, and as she was a woman and had been in the public eye, what she wrote attracted attention. But, for all her struggle and success, she was still a young and inexperienced practitioner, qualified for a year only after a desultory training during which the last subject likely to have been studied was venereal disease. If she had been older or wiser she would have kept out of this battle, but the suggestion that she supported the Contagious Diseases Acts for an unworthy motive, such as gaining favour with her medical confrères, will be dismissed by all who appreciate her character, and need not be discussed. The campaign led by Mrs. Butler and growing doubt of the efficacy of the measures led to the repeal of the Acts in 1886. Later, in 1891 at the Hygienic Congress, the medical profession condemned the regulations as useless.

By 1869 Miss Garrett's private practice had grown considerably and it and her work at the St. Mary's Dispensary kept her busy. When, however, a vacancy occurred on the honorary medical staff of the Shadwell Hospital for Children (now the Princess Elizabeth of York Hospital for Children) she applied for the post. Dr. John Murray and Mr. Heckford who were on the staff of the hospital were her friends. Dr. Murray's acquaintance dated from her student days at the Middlesex Hospital; and Mr. Heckford, who was a member of

The Paris M.D.

the consulting staff of the London Hospital, had helped
Elizabeth during her difficulties there.

Miss Garrett was on the selected list and accordingly
was interviewed by the board, one of whose members,
J. G. S. Anderson, has left his impression on record.
His firm, a shipping business in the city, contributed to
the hospital funds and he was a member of the board as
their representative. He had not intended to support
Miss Garrett's application but after watching her and
listening to her replies, he had done so. She was successful and, after the meeting ended, Mr. Anderson and she
had a short conversation. 'I caught her as she was going
downstairs,' he said. He told her that one of his sisters
thought of studying medicine. This was interesting. Also
Miss Garrett discovered that Dr. John Murray was his
cousin and Dr. J. Ford Anderson, an acquaintance at the
Middlesex Hospital, his brother. Before many weeks
passed Miss Garrett was appointed a medical representative on the Board of Management of the hospital. She,
Dr. Murray and Mr. Anderson agreed that the adminis-
tration might be improved and they worked together
to bring about reforms. During 1869 letters on Shadwell
Hospital business passed frequently between Miss Garrett and Mr. Anderson and they became friendly.

Although she had been in practice for four years, Miss
Garrett decided to take the Paris M.D. degree if she
could obtain permission to sit for the examinations without living in Paris as a student, otherwise she meant to

try one of the German universities. The University of Paris opened its medical degree to women in 1868 and Miss Garrett was the first woman to avail herself of this concession. A foreign degree would not be recognized by the British Medical Register, but as supplementary to the licence of the Apothecaries' Hall Society she knew that it would be worth having. At this stage in her life it was an undertaking to face six examinations in a foreign language. She was not a linguist; by this time she was extremely busy and examinations become tiresome after the age of thirty.

To relearn the preliminary subjects, such as chemistry and anatomy, was fatiguing, but by dint of early rising and working as she drove to see her patients, she prepared for the examinations. One afternoon when the bones of the disjointed skeleton were scattered over the table, the door was thrown open and the maid announced, 'Her Royal Highness, the Princess Louise' A pleasant visit followed and Elizabeth, taking a roseate view of royalty, treasured every word the Princess uttered. Rumour said that Queen Victoria disapproved of the visit, made without her knowledge; at any rate it was not repeated. 'I am glad the Princess Louise takes an interest,' wrote Mrs. Russell Gurney and added a blessing, 'Strength and Peace to you.'

Lord Lyons, British Ambassador in Paris, helped Elizabeth to secure permission to sit before the examining board of the Paris University without living in

The Paris M.D.

Paris, and also acted as emissary of the Emperor Napoleon III, from whom he gave her a friendly message.

Altogether she visited Paris six times, and in quick succession and with distinction passed each of the six examinations. While in Paris Elizabeth boarded with the family of one of the professors of the Sorbonne, feeling happy in the academic society to which she was introduced. This is a story of that period. At a party she made an assertion and a Frenchman said 'How like an English woman!' 'That is the last thing I mind being called,' the visitor replied. In rapid French, with gesticulation, he said, 'No wonder we dislike you. Now if you said to me, "How like a Frenchman!" it would not be a compliment at all. I should feel humiliated, but with you it is different. I say "How British!" and you are pleased. It is annoying.'

By June 1870 she was ready to take the final M.D. Before starting she wrote:

E.G. to J.G.S.A.   *3 June 1870*
'My Paris summons came this morning. Drink to my becoming a great physician on the 15th with 30 years of vigour before one; surely this is not too much to look for?'

The good wishes of many friends went with her but none pleased her more than the message from Mrs. Russell Gurney.

The Paris M.D.

Mrs. Russell Gurney to E.G.   *15 June 1870*

'Your dear note has only just reached me as I was detained unexpectedly in the country and my letters were not forwarded. But tho' I was not in time to answer and have a glimpse of you before you went I can now follow you in thought and rejoice with you and look up with large desires and hopes for you—my dear, dear one—and I have some conviction that your (*our* I may say) beloved one is also with us in thought and hope. How you have been prospered and how you have worked and willed since I saw you as a bud 10 years ago—was it? Now the fowls of the air may lodge in your branches. May your roots be ever directed to the Water of Life more and more so that shade and healing and fruit may come thro' you to many people. Please offer my warmest congratulations to your happy Father and Mother.'

Her thesis was on 'La Migraine'. In the *viva voce* examination which followed the examiners took her to task for her ignorance of the distinction of Dr. Graves of Dublin: 'Mademoiselle, vous ne connaissez pas donc vos grands hommes.' 'Mais, monsieur,' she replied, 'nous en avons tant,' whereat they laughed and forgave her. A few days later she wrote to tell Mr. J. G. S. Anderson that she had passed: 'Wednesday's business went well enough and I am now M.D.' The Medical Press, especially the *British Medical Journal* under the editorship of Dr. Ernest Hart, was extremely cordial about Elizabeth's successes in Paris, and the *Lancet* records: 'Her friends must have been highly gratified to hear how her judges congratulated her on her success and to see what sympathy and respect was shown to her by all present.' To a friend Elizabeth wrote: 'In spite of all this [praise] E.G. does not when she is free to be candid think much of herself.'

By this time under the leadership of Miss Sophia Jex-Blake, six women were studying medicine in Edinburgh and they wrote to Miss Garrett to congratulate her on taking the Paris degree.

S.J.-B. and others to E.G.   *Edinburgh, 20 June 1870*
'We cannot refrain from offering you our hearty congratulations on the brilliant success at Paris which has at length crowned your many years of arduous work— work whose difficulties perhaps no one can estimate so well as ourselves. And while congratulating you on receiving the highest honours of your profession from one of the first medical schools in the world, we desire to express also our appreciation of the example you have afforded to others, and the honour you have reflected on all women who have chosen medicine as their profession.'

They also wrote to the *Pall Mall Gazette* a letter which pleased her.

The Paris M.D.

E.G. to J.G.S.A.   *23 June 1870*

'If you see the *Pall Mall* look out for a charming little
letter from the Edinburgh students to me. It gave me a
great deal of pleasure, it was so kind of them to think of
it, and one's artistic sense was gratified by their saying
exactly what it is pleasant to have said in the way of
congratulation.'

E.G. to J.G.S.A.   *30 June 1870*

'You hit the nail on the head when you said you would
not have known my style in the answer to the Edinburgh
students. The difference of style one falls quite naturally
into in writing a formal letter which is probably meant
to last is as great as the difference between fireside gossip
and a public speech. I think the gossip need not be dated
and "turned" and that the speech ought to be both.'

Side by side with Elizabeth's professional work went
the campaign for the parliamentary enfranchisement of
women. She did not speak at suffrage meetings nor take
a prominent part in their organization, thinking it would
be unwise to become identified with a second unpopular
cause. Nevertheless, she gave her whole-hearted adher-
ence. Lady Amberley gives an account of one of these
early meetings.

Diary of Lady Amberley (from the Amberley Papers)
26 March 1870

'The meeting of the Women's Suffrage Society had

134

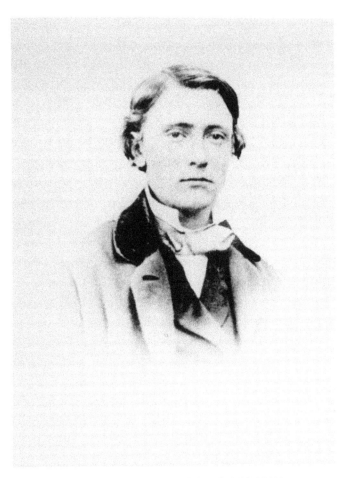

J. G. S. ANDERSON AS A YOUNG MAN

been fixed for to-day partly to suit Amberley as he was to speak, so he had to go in spite of his neuralgia but he felt very ill indeed. The meeting was in the Hanover Square Rooms—I sat on the platform in front between A. and Miss Taylor. The room was very full of well-dressed people. . . . Miss Taylor made a long and much studied speech; it was good but too like acting. Mrs. Grote's was short but natural—Mrs. Fawcett's uninteresting and Mrs. Pet Taylor (Chairman) was inaudible from sore throat. It went off very well and was a great success.'

The conversion of Mrs. Grote to the enfranchisement of women took place about the time of J. S. Mill's petition. She had been robbed of her purse and in the police court it was described as the property of Mr. Grote. Most indignant, she exclaimed: 'When I discovered that the purse in my pocket and the watch at my side were not my own but the Historian's, I felt it was time women should have the power to amend these preposterous laws.' In 1877 a similar experience occurred to Mrs. Fawcett [Millicent Garrett]. On the charge sheet was written, 'Stealing from the person of Millicent Fawcett a purse containing £1.18.6 the property of Henry Fawcett.' The thief was sentenced to seven years' penal servitude—a terrible sentence compared with the one he would receive to-day.

Elizabeth has left no comment on Mrs. Grote's appearance. She was a valuable ally and greatly respected. However, Sidney Smith's remarks may be remembered. 'At last I know the meaning of the word grotesque,' as Mrs. Grote in a pink turban entered the drawing-room; also his question about her: 'Who is the gentleman in white muslin on the sofa?'

By 1870 Miss Garrett's private practice was steadily increasing, and she constantly met in consultation the leading physicians in London. Her choice of consultant usually fell on one of the physicians from the Middlesex Hospital with whom she established most cordial relations. An impression of the effect she had on her patients is given in a letter from Mrs. Russell Gurney. 'Dear Goddess of Health,' she wrote, 'you brought in with you such a fresh current of health and vigour that you took away my cold and I perceived a *radiance* for some time afterwards.'

6

INTERLUDES 1870
FRANCO-PRUSSIAN WAR
FIRST LONDON SCHOOL
BOARD ELECTION

⪻⪻⪼●⪻⪻⪻

When, in the summer of 1870, war between France and Germany broke out, Elizabeth's sympathy was with the French.

E.G. to J.G.S.A.   *10 Aug. 1870*
'It is sadly difficult even to pretend to do anything but read the papers and look at the map.'

A few days later Elizabeth wrote again to Mr. Anderson about the hospital, where arrangements were not to her liking.

E.G. to J.G.S.A.   *20 Aug. 1870*
'Unless we are tolerably well satisfied with the way in which it is worked it is better to leave it and turn to some other equally useful little charity more to our taste than to waste time and temper in endless efforts to put things straight. I am not benevolent, there is not time to be everything and I put that *rôle* aside along with hundreds of others. It is my business to become a great physician, nothing else I could do would help women

137

so much as this, therefore if the hospital helps it is welcome, if it hinders away with it! I never felt so sure of
the good of war[1] as now when one has no words for
one's sympathy with France. It is a great thing to be
alive just now and to have such an experience first hand.
Reading even about Marathon will be tame by comparison for ever after it. How I wish Tennyson would
put our inarticulate awe as witnesses of this tragedy into
words, solemn and thrilling enough to stir our children
and to show them what this month has been to us.'

London day by day was placarded with the news of
great battles in which the Germans were victorious and
the French defeated with terrible casualties. Some of her
friends, among them Mr. Norton, the surgeon, were
serving with the French Red Cross.

Elizabeth had a few days' leisure and she suggested
taking her undergraduate brother Sam, and her sister
Josephine, aged eighteen, to Brussels. Perhaps they might
see for themselves what was going on, at any rate a short
holiday abroad would be pleasant after her hard work.
Before starting she wrote to Mr. Anderson. By this time
she regarded him as a friend as well as a colleague, hence
the little joke about the dangers of an out-patient department.

E.G. to J.G.S.A.   *London, 5 Sept. 1870*
'I never make light of an ally, nor do I persist in doing

[1] probably by stimulating courage and self-sacrifice.

his work as well as my own. *Ergo* I sail for Antwerp at noon to-morrow. But your work at the Committee will not be hard, as our advice is given with overpowering unanimity. Dr. Walker stood out a little against my proposal to fix the patient's chair to the floor, but as he gleefully owned that fleas were nothing to him, his less happy confrères were allowed to carry their point. I am not going on an errand of mercy, though if I could talk German I should have been glad to do so. One of my brothers will join me at Antwerp and our plan is to get down to the frontier and then act as prudence may suggest.'

The holiday-makers had no misgiving about the propriety of sightseeing in a war zone. They enjoyed their strange trip; during which Elizabeth wrote three letters in pencil, on scraps of paper. Extracts from those to her father and Mr. Anderson follow.

E.G. to N.G.   *On the road from Arlon to Sedan,*
12 Sept. 1870

'It was very late when we reached Arlon. However we found quarters. The only drawback to the inn was a terrible smell of drains in our room, it was horrible. Having the fear of gastric fever before our eyes, we slept with our heads wrapped in Shetland shawls with three folds over our mouths to keep out the stench. We have no luggage and very little money with us as we were afraid of robbers.'

139

Interludes 1870

E.G. to J.G.S.A.   *On an ambulance waggon from*
Bouillon to Sedan, 12 Sept. 1870

'I think you will perhaps like a note from this novel position. Anyhow having 4 hours on my hands I shall like to write. To make the position clear I must go back a little. My companions, a young brother of 20 and a still younger sister, met me at Antwerp and from Thursday to Sunday we were doing the ordinary deeds of tourists—opera every night and so on. Yesterday we left for Arlon. On the road we met an ambulance train. It was a sight one does not quickly forget. At a quiet country station in the bright moonlight rows of stretchers on the ground being carefully lifted into the carriages. . . . We had counted on having dinner at Bouillon and then getting a carriage to Sedan but we found it impossible to get even a biscuit and quite impossible to get even the promise of a horse for to-morrow or of beds. At the barracks the Prussian officer allowed us to sit in one of the ambulance waggons going back to Sedan with stores for the hospital. Captain in first waggon, we in second, then 11 others trailing along at foot pace. At last by moonlight entering the gates of Sedan at 11.30 p.m. We had unwillingly to turn out of our waggon and begin our search for rooms. Every hotel was full and we began to be in despair. Found a church open with one lamp alight, peeped in saw a bier with a dead man on it and thought we would not lodge there. Clocks now striking 12. Here our adventures became so serious that I must ask you to consider them confidential. Saw an officer—thought he looked good and rushed at him with our anxieties—learning that we had tried all the hotels he asked us home with him, saying that J. and I could have his room. This morning we found our good Samaritan had passed the night on a chair. On the return journey by train at a small station we waited 3-4 hours spending the time distributing chocolate and tobacco, water and apples to the wounded. My sister is particularly good at this sort of work as she is pretty enough to be a reviving attendant. And at 18 there is a charm in the smallest action of kindliness. "Madame votre mère", as the soldiers named me in conversing with their favourite, contented herself with the more prosaic work of dressing their wounds. Not being able to get to Metz we are now coming homewards.'

None of the letters mentioned the present bought for the kind Prussian officer. After the night at Sedan in his room the three young people had counted their money —a small store unfortunately owing to fear of 'robbers' —and had scraped together enough to buy him a diamond ring as a memento. It was a handsome stone set in a dog collar of gold—no doubt diamonds were cheap in Sedan at such a time. Even so, to buy a diamond at all was a new experience to them, and their eagerness to present this splendid thank-offering can be imagined. Picture their distress as each expected the other to remember in what street the officer lodged, and to what regiment he belonged, and what was his name. But as none of them could answer any of the questions they were never able to thank their kind host and I now wear the diamond.

The German advance was rapid and the siege of Paris began shortly after Elizabeth's party reached home. Foreigners were allowed to leave the city and among the refugees two American women escaped to London. They felt ill and they were friendless. Miss Garrett, whom they consulted, diagnosed incipient small-pox. As no state hospitals for infectious disease existed and as no lodgings would receive them, she put these complete strangers to bed in the upper floor of her house where they recovered and became her devoted friends. Such interludes varied the routine of an increasingly busy life.

About this time Miss Garrett began to work closely with Mr. Anderson in an effort to improve organization in the Shadwell Hospital. The board meetings of the hospital were held at the City office of Mr. Anderson's firm in Lime Street Square and many letters passed between them on this business. Mr. Anderson was an officer in the London Scottish and during the summer (1870) his regiment was under canvas at Wimbledon. He asked Miss Garrett to visit him there; and in July, accompanied by Miss Emily Davies, she went, taking a copy of Wordsworth's poems to read aloud if the occasion arose. Mr. Anderson welcomed the ladies—a handsome gracious host in his uniform of 'hodden grey' with all its Scottish finery. After this outing Miss Davies wrote with uncommon tact, 'of all your friends I like Mr. Anderson the best!' In return for his hospitality, Miss Garrett occasionally asked him to dinner. Miss Jane Crowe who lived with her would be present but that was not enough, and she always had 'a party' when he came. She tried to provide good company for him and even to ensure that he should shine among her other guests, inculcating the art of general conversation.

E.G. to J.G.S.A.   *London, 23 Oct. 1870*

'I wonder if I may venture to be that odious person, "a candid friend", and tell you of a flaw I saw in you as guest last night? I will risk it, for I know you will be grateful when you have digested my criticism. I perceived that you did not know that the centre guest along the line of the table has the post of difficulty as far as talking goes. If he whispers to his neighbours general talk is impossible; his duty is plain—to talk to the Chair or rather to the two Chairs—he ought to be the link between the two ends, the most useful of guests, if he sees his true importance. It is curious how few people know this element in the art of social talk. I saw it years ago and am quite distressed with a sense of bad generalship when my centres turn out inefficient. Can you forgive me? Miss Cobbe, Sir Henry and Lady Thompson, Professor Beesly and some artists will be here next

Saturday. If you would come in at 9.30 I think you would like them and I should understand that you do not bear malice.'

He had evidently been talking to his neighbours and not to her—which was tactless, one must admit, when they were on the terms this letter and its reception indicate. That he did not bear malice is shown in a pencil note from her two days later, written driving. 'I am grateful to you for not being vexed,' she says. Gradually she learnt more about him. He was a born story-teller. His father, the Rev. Alexander Anderson, at that time a schoolmaster at Chanonry, Old Aberdeen, had been a minister in the Established Church of Scotland until, in the Great Disruption of 1843, he and four hundred others had thrown up their livings as a protest against patronage in the appointments to the ministry.

In those days a minister in a good living in Scotland was one of the well-to-do members of a simple society. Dr. Anderson and his wife had had a comfortable house and a staff of servants. Then, on a point of conscience, their income ceased and they lost their home. The maids had to be paid off, but Annie Peters, the nurse, and Jane Day, the cook, refused to go. They preferred to remain without wages. Presently Dr. Anderson was called to another 'charge' and comfort and a home returned. Within a short time Dr. Anderson differed from his church about total immersion at baptism and, as a result, his wife and family were penniless and homeless again. At this second crisis as at the first, Annie Peters stood firm—her duty was to look after her bairns, and pay or no pay, food or less food, she would stay with the family. Jane Day however said she must look after herself and so, with tears, she left. After a week's absence, with more tears and still no pay, she returned. These dear friends remained with the family until they died, sixty years later, but Annie Peters never forgot that week of absence. Jane Day to her remained the 'newcomer'.

James George was five at the Great Disruption. He forgot nothing: the day was wet; they left the manse in carts; they were boarded out among the fisher folk of Whitehills on the bleak Aberdeenshire coast. After this Mrs. Anderson suggested that her husband should find work which put less strain on his conscience; he took the hint and started a school for boys—the Gymnasium at Chanonry, Old Aberdeen, the first school of its quality in Scotland. Distinguished men issued from it to glorify 'Guvvie's' name and, for half a century, they toasted him and their old school in remote corners of the world. From the Gymnasium an income flowed in, and Dr. Anderson was able to start eleven children in life. James George, the second son, was educated at the village school, Whitehills, by his father and at the Universities of Aberdeen and Bonn. Through this varied curriculum he sped so fast that at sixteen he accepted the invitation

of his uncle James Anderson to come to London to the
shipping firm of George Thomson & Co. The young
man did not spring into wealth. He started on a salary
of two pounds a week from which a small contribution
was sent home. As his earnings increased a brother and
sister were confided to his care and at his own expense
he fitted out little Nellie (later Mrs. Auckland Geddes)
for her first boarding-school and chose her hats, which
he found difficult. When Miss Garrett made the acquaintance of J. G. S. Anderson he was a man of thirty
regarded as a confirmed bachelor.

In less than a year a new and unexpected develop-
ment brought them together in even closer co-operation than the work they had shared for the hospital.
Women were admitted to the municipal franchise in
1869 and the following year new opportunities were
opened to them by Mr. Forster's Education Act, under
which they gained the right not only to vote but to
stand for election to the School Board.

The Act created a complete system of elementary
education, with school boards specially elected as education authorities. It was an immensely important piece of
legislation destined to alter the character of the English
people. Four women presented themselves as candidates.
Flora Stevenson in Edinburgh, Lydia Becker in Manchester, Emily Davies in Greenwich and, in response to
a deputation from the husbands of her patients at the
dispensary, Elizabeth Garrett in Marylebone. The invita-

tion reached her officially from a Working Men's Association in the Marylebone Division and she lost no time in writing to Miss Davies.

E.G. to E.D.   *London, 24 Oct. 1870*

'This morning I had a deputation from working men. They think there must be meetings to teach people to be interested. I suppose it is part of the whole thing and ought not to be refused tho' I am sorry it is so. I dare say when it has to be done I can do it, and it is no use asking for women to be taken into public work and yet to wish them to avoid publicity. We must be ready to go into the thing as men do if we go at all. Still I am very sorry it is necessary, especially as I can't think of anything to say for four speeches! and after Huxley too, who speaks in epigrams! The first of these trials is to be next week. Bless us, it is a tough and toilsome business.'

An election committee consisting of many well-known residents in Marylebone was formed in addition to that of the Working Men's Association.

Miss Garrett's supporters included the Rev. S. A. Barnett, Mme Bodichon, Miss Buss, Dr. Andrew Clark, Leonard Courtney, the Rev. J. Ll. Davies, Professor Fawcett, V. H. Flower, F.R.S., the Rev. H. R. Haweis, Octavia Hill, the Rev. W. J. Loftie, Professor Masson, Sir Frederick Pollock, Norman Lockyer, the Hon. Mr. Justice Hannen, Professor Adams, Charlton Bastian, F.R.S., Julia Wedgewood, Sir Henry Thompson, Henry

Sidgwick—names which suggest a panorama of the period and of the women's movement. Mr. Robert Browning proved an active worker in the election campaign but he did not join the committee.

By a slight manœuvre Miss Garrett secured the appointment of the officers she thought best for her committee. She wrote to a member before an early meeting of the executive.

E.G. to Mrs. Jackson   *Undated*
'I have had an idea. How would it do to depose Mr. Christie from the executive, leaving him still chairman of the general committee, put Mr. Anderson in his place and let him give all the orders to Mr. Hill. I feel very much that we need a better head to the executive, the meetings are pretty much waste of time as they are now conducted.

'Will you please confer with Mrs. Westlake over this and let me know your two opinions. Mr. Anderson is quite to be trusted in all questions that require decision, energy and sound sense.' A postscript was added:

'Mr. C. has resigned very good-humouredly. Will you please move that Mr. Anderson take the chair, permanently, at the executive? He agrees to this.'

The chairman coached and advised the candidate and he wrote the leaflet pressing her claims on the ratepayers, each of whom had as many votes as there were members to be elected. The votes could be divided or concentrated on one candidate. Across the draft leaflet the chairman wrote, 'cut and carve to your own liking getting it first copied out in a roomy way'. The Press was sympathetic.

At this date women seldom appeared on public platforms and speeches were considered the province of men. It was usual to ask 'a gentleman' to read a woman's speech. But a popular election demanded more than this from the candidate, and Elizabeth found herself addressing audiences constantly in halls and out of doors. The practice was invaluable. Sometimes she was heckled but she was courageous and honest and her answers won support. She was not an orator and her voice was unsuited to large halls but she became a reliable and ready speaker.

In addition to speaking in her own division she went to Greenwich to support the candidature of Miss Emily Davies, who wrote to a friend on 25 November, 'I cannot help wishing you had been at Greenwich. You would have liked Miss Garrett's speech—it was only too generous—and the meeting was enthusiastic. The hall was fuller than it would hold (it holds 1,000) and the women came crowding into the Committee Room at the end to shake hands and to promise their votes.'[1] As Mr. Anderson was both chairman of her election committee and her colleague on the Board of the Shadwell Hospital, Miss Garrett was obliged to write to him often.

[1] Reprinted from *Emily Davies and Girton College* by Barbara Stephen.

Interludes 1870

'Would it not save trouble if I sent you £100 to go on
with so that bills could be paid immediately? I hate debts
and paying directly would not encourage extravagance
but rather the contrary. Miss Davies, my one clear-
sighted, critical and honest friend who knows me thro'
and thro' and entirely without glamour (every one else
has either imperfect knowledge or glamour), will keep
me from putting any too daring untruths into the paper.
It would be effective if you could bear testimony to my
having been of use to a committee of men. It is not
unlike what the School Board work will be and requires
the same qualities. That you were against me [when she
applied for the hospital post] makes your testimony the
more valuable.' As an afterthought she wrote: 'Don't
think I am against glamour. Life would be insupportable
without it, much as I appreciate its absence in one
friend.'

The district to be canvassed was large. It included
Hampstead and St. Pancras as well as Marylebone. A
public meeting held on 11 November in St. George's
Hall roused much support. As the contest went on the
chairman thought the candidate received injudicious and
excessive praise and wrote to warn her of its bad effects.

E.G. to J.G.S.A.   *London, 13 Nov. 1870*

'I have been pondering over your terrible hint as to
the effects of butter. I thought about it while it was going

on and decided that so long as it was not swallowed and absorbed it could not do much harm. I *do* rejoice in every gift however trifling that makes me more fit for the special niche I am meant to fill but I don't think this really hurts me. The corrective is found in not living a self-concentrated life, in caring for great things and in an enthusiasm of admiration for those before whom oneself is pigmied. It is only in Lilliput Land that I could be stuck-up and thank Heaven I am not living there yet, tho' one does occasionally meet one of its inhabitants and think much of oneself in consequence.'

She addressed some midday meetings of workmen in their dinner hour. Her audiences were of many trades and she had to overcome some prejudice. Postcards to her chairman reported progress.

E.G. to J.G.S.A.　　　　　*London, 16 Nov. 1870*
'A most enthusiastic workmen's meeting to-night. An important vestryman knocked under completely and begged me to take Grafton Hall in the Tottenham Court Road for one night next week. The vestryman convert, who is by profession an undertaker, will preside.'

Two days later she wrote:

E.G. to J.G.S.A.　　　　　*London, 18 Nov. 1870*
'Collards' have invited me to address their employees to-morrow at 2. There are 600 of them, all earning from 30/- to £3.10.0 per week.'

Interludes 1870

By this time her distaste for publicity had waned and she was able to enjoy the campaign.

E.G. to J.G.S.A.   *London, 20 Nov. 1870*

'The open-air meeting of Collards' men went very well. It was delightfully picturesque. I did not stand on a barrel as I had feared might have been the plan, but on some steps leading from a balcony into the yard. About 300 men and boys were there, one man spoke very well for me at the end of the affair.'

During the last days of the contest the usual anxiety showed itself.

E.G. to J.G.S.A.   *London, Nov. 1870*

'I am not satisfied that we are doing enough, or planning to do so, for this last week. Large districts are still untouched from want of canvassers. Would it be possible for you to dine with us at 6 to-night as the only chance of discussing other schemes with me? I am very busy all to-day and shall not be at home till just before 6 o'clock. The Eyre Arms meeting was scarcely a success. I was much dissatisfied with my own share in the performance.'

That the candidate did not always consult her chairman is seen from the following letter which suggests that some religious question was at stake.

J.G.S.A. to E.G.   *London, 24 Nov. 1870*

'I am heart-broken at the step you have taken. You

152

have lost yourself thousands of votes, and you have taken the guidance of your affairs out of the hands of your committee, and you have shewn as you say weakness and vacillation. It was most unfortunate. Christie is a bad counsellor. His injudicious enlargement upon pietists and religionists at St. George's Hall shewed me that he did not recognize the forces on which we have to rely.'

In Elizabeth's reply to this outburst she confessed herself at fault but warned him not to be long-winded in addressing one of the final meetings.

E.G. to J.G.S.A.   *London, 24 Nov. 1870*

'I don't think you could say anything more useful or effective than what you have already said for me. An actual bit of experience tells so well. It might perhaps be said rather more shortly, I thought it would have been more entertaining if somewhat condensed but I know I have an almost morbid love of brevity. Suppose you say nothing about the Mansion House meeting which was really a mere trifle, and bring out distinctly that a committee of City men had found me useful and not insufferably disagreeable. Please don't call me energetic (I am ready to wish I were indolent by way of change) and I should dislike any one extremely whose chief recommendation was energy and in a woman it is peculiarly unattractive. It suggests hurry and bustle and strangers would not know that I was not a prey to these vices.'

Interludes 1870

The election results were published late on 30 November.

E.G. to J.G.S.A.   *London, 30 Nov. 1870*

'You will get the news from the evening papers probably as early as I do, as I have some long rounds to go this afternoon and shall miss any special message sent to me. Edmund [her brother] will have told you, or left word, the result of the 12 divisions counted up at 6 o'clock. Unless the others are very different the victory is complete. I am very glad and happy, both for the victory itself and also for it having been given to me to have a share in it. I am sure it will do the women's cause great good. I wish very much that I could find some adequate way of thanking you and all my other zealous friends. But I am quite beggared. I can find no words that do not seem either too small or too common or too formal. It is not however difficult to me to take help of any kind from friends, it does not burden me so long as I know I would do as much for them, or more if I could, and for the others I suppose one ought to be humble enough not to feel very much oppressed, tho' I admit that poor Mr. Hay Hill will seem like a creditor for whom one has none of the right coin, to the rest of my days.'

E.G. to J.G.S.A.   Post Card, 12 p.m., 30 Nov. 1870

Garrett	47,848
Huxley	13,494

Interludes 1870

Thorold	12,186
Angus	11,472
Hutchins	9,253
Dixon	9,031
Watson	8,355

The School Board election results were a stupendous victory for the women's cause. All the women candidates had been returned and Miss Garrett's 47,848 votes were the largest number won by any candidate at the election. She and her supporters could not help noticing with pride that Professor Huxley, great man as he was, had made a poor show as second on the list, epigrams notwithstanding. Even in the turmoil of victory, snowed under by congratulations and obliged to write innumerable letters to those who had worked for her, Elizabeth Garrett had time to correct grammatical errors from her chairman.

E.G. to J.G.S.A.   *2 Dec. 1870*
'*Shall and Will.* Observe that both words may mean either prediction or volition. "Shall" used by the first person, singular or plural, predicts only: used by the 2nd or 3rd person, it expresses *volition only* (examples are not needed for intelligent scholars). The converse of the rule for "shall" governs the use of "will", which in the first person means volition, in the 2nd and 3rd prediction. A more difficult thing would be to explain how it is that Scotch people don't know these two words by

the light of nature. It is queer too how we come to use them in this puzzling and reverse method.'

E.G. to J.G.S.A.   *3 Dec. 1870*
'I wrote yesterday a hurried but brief note to my 86 St. Pancras, 35 Paddington and 15 Hampstead workers. Heaven grant that they do not think they require an answer! My maid wonders how I can ever read those I have now and "to answer them, Ma'am!" I agree with her and am counting on "no postman" to-morrow.'

E.G. to J.G.S.A.   *4 Dec. 1870*
'I heard yesterday of a plumper given by a man who had never spoken to me but had seen me once in a new gown at a party. For the gown's sake only he voted. And then women are thought to be unfit for the franchise!'

The first meeting of the newly appointed London School Board was to take place in the Guildhall. Elizabeth wondered whether she, as the recipient of the largest number of votes, should take the chair if offered to her, pending the election of the permanent chairman.

E.G. to J.G.S.A.   *6 Dec. 1870*
'I have been with the Recorder and Mrs. Russell Gurney this evening. They are so happy over our victory and they think it a grand step towards the franchise. They find it "taxes their affection not to be shy with

such a conqueror". They are quite strongly in favour of my taking the chair the first day.'

Miss Davies on the other hand was horrified at the suggestion.

E.D. to E.G.   *London, 7 Dec. 1870*

'The temporary chair question does not seem to be very important. I was a little sorry that you should tell people, whether in jest or earnest, that you would very much like a position which to my mind, would be incongruous even to the point of absurdity. I should feel it so in my own case, tho' as the Scotsman observed, I am "of comparatively mature age" and have had more experience of that sort. It is not being a woman (tho' that probably enhances it) but your youth and inexperience that makes it strike me as almost indecorous to think of presiding over men like Lord Lawrence [recent Viceroy of India], etc. It may not strike others in the same way, and if there were a rule, it might be worth while to submit to it, but there can scarcely be precedents enough to constitute a custom, and unless necessary, I should be sorry for you to do anything which might give colour to the charge of being "cheeky", which has been brought against you lately. It is too true that your jokes are many and reckless. They do more harm than you know.'

The letter ended with a friendly reference to Mr. Anderson and Elizabeth sent it to him.

Interludes 1870

'Most people like compliments, particularly when they have the charm of perfect sincerity, so I send you one from Miss Davies. Miss Davies is a good deal my senior and if I live to be 100 she will still be so and will feel it as much as she did when I sat at her feet in girlhood. I enjoy thinking how I can crush her with the Recorder's and Mrs. Russell Gurney's decided opinion on the other side. I ought to have been luminous in the dark last night, I had been dining with such a constellation, Robert Browning, Jenny Lind, Dean Stanley and Lady Augusta and Professor Mohl. It was very delightful to be thought fit for such companions. Lady Augusta sees all the advantages our victory brings to the general cause and rejoices over them very cordially. (I decided as I talked to her that she was the first person of quite superior intelligence and sweet manner I had ever noticed with a long upper lip.) I was sorry to see nothing of you last night, but the room was full of friends who demanded a word.'

The question of the temporary chairmanship had been decided before Miss Davies and Miss Garrett reached the Guildhall.

E.G. to J.G.S.A.   *London, 15 Dec. 1870*

'I had no choice about the chair, after all! It had evidently been arranged beforehand that I should have none. When we assembled Miss Davies and I were asked to take two seats apart, this we resisted and with the Recorder's sanction sat on a level with the other members on the seat round the table facing the House. Without a moment's pause some one moved that the oldest member should take the chair; then some one amended it that Aldn. Cotton should. It was seconded and carried without discussion. After a few commonplaces from him, Huxley opened the battle by moving that *no* salary be given to the chairman. (We had arranged last night that this should be the procedure as a negative could be moved without notice.) To my surprise most people agreed to the no salary principle, Lord Sandon, Dr. Barry, Mr. Thorold and Mr. Smith were all on our side. They said nearly all I had thought of, but as I thought it would look less like being sore about the chairmanship to say a word or two in a good-humoured way, I just added that I heartily supported Mr. Huxley's motion—without giving reasons. Then we voted and it passed by 32 to 14. It is curiously like Parliament. We admitted strangers, so you must come and see us some day. It was very pleasant to Miss Davies and me to have the Recorder's friendly presence all the time. I felt the atmosphere to be decidedly hostile, but of course that is not surprising and it is not a bad discipline to find it so after the intoxication of one's 47,000. The anteroom was full of my supporters who gave me a hearty welcome as I came in.'

159

Interludes 1870

One of Miss Garrett's admirers without her knowledge published an appeal for funds to pay her election expenses. The terms of this appeal—in fact an appeal at all—was distasteful to her. 'He will make me a byword among beggars if we do not stop him,' she wrote.

E.G. to J.G.S.A.   *London, 16 Dec. 1870*

'I have written to say I wish nothing more to be done in the way of getting money and that the accounts are to be put into your hands on Monday in order that I may settle them with you before leaving London for Christmas. Another bill for printing (£15) I send to Mr. Slader to-day. Even with this, the deficit will not be much over £100, a very moderate price to pay for so high a pinnacle! *The Times* and the *Daily News* both report yesterday's meeting very well. I was sorry afterwards I said so little, but I was really a little awed by the whole thing being so extremely like Parliament and by having to spring up so quickly to get a hearing after some one else had finished. The whole difficulty of speaking is concentrated in that moment of swift self-assertion.'

The delight of Elizabeth Garrett in her election was shared by others. 'I am much pleased at Miss Garrett's success,' wrote Lord Russell, ex-Prime Minister, to Lord Amberley, 'she ought to have a vote for Westminster, but not to sit in Parliament. It would make too much confusion.' (*Amberley Papers.*)

Interludes 1870

A contemporary painting of the meeting of the first London School Board hangs in the County Hall, Westminster. It may not be a masterpiece but it serves as a memorial of an interesting and important event. The success of the women candidates not only strengthened the women's movement but helped Elizabeth Garrett as its missioner in her profession. It launched her as a personage in exactly the society she and her cause needed. She was an attraction to hostesses and her social engagements were numerous and exciting.

E.G. to J.G.S.A.   *London, 21 Dec. 1870*

'I have been to the artist Armitage's to-night and have met Sant, Wells and plenty of French dons. I am above par just now, so I am eating an unwholesome number of good dinners. Now I have to consider how I can cover myself in a cloak of darkness and run out to the post with this. Certainly in the matter of clothes we women are heavily weighted. I often envy the wearers of dress-coats, so changeless and so easy to hide and walk out in.'

E. G. to J.G.S.A.   *London, 23 Dec. 1870*

'I shall be at home this evening but *perhaps* it would be better for you not to come. I should not like to confuse my maid's sense of decorum and I am afraid it might. Since writing this some photos have come from Caldesi's on which I will extract an opinion the next time I see you. They are less repulsive I think than any done before, but one does not judge well for oneself. Caldesi is anxious to sell them. I have always refused, but if either of these is creditable it might perhaps save trouble and give some people a little pleasure to allow it. Perhaps you might compromise with Mrs. Grundy if you come to-night by not staying so long?'

He acted on the suggestion but whether he compromised with Mrs. Grundy is uncertain. At any rate, the visit was long enough to allow matters to be settled between them. They became engaged, and it was decided that they should go to Aldeburgh the following day in order to introduce Jamie to Mr. and Mrs. Garrett and to the rest of the family assembled there for the Christmas holidays. Elizabeth arranged to go by an early train and he would follow later. Perhaps she thought the interval before his arrival might be spent in reconciling her family, especially Mr. Garrett, to her engagement.

7

ENGAGEMENT

>>⊃●⊂<<

In December 1870 Miss Garrett's engagement to Mr.
James George Skelton Anderson, shipowner, was announced. The news created widespread interest. Letters
poured in and the one that pleased her most was from
Miss Davies. Knowing Elizabeth 'through and through'
it did not occur to her as it did to others that she would
desert the cause or forsake her profession. She wrote
with tenderness, understanding and complete unselfish-
ness.

    E.D. to E.G.   *24 Dec. 1870*

'I don't think you either foolish or selfish and I rejoice
with a full heart. Do you remember my saying to you
a little while ago that I liked him the best of all your
friends? I meant you to understand that I was ready to
be glad, but perhaps it was not strong enough to strike
you. I don't know how I could have endured it if you
had married anybody whom I could not heartily respect
as well as like. It is very sweet to me to be able to be so

happy about it. It does not make me feel as if I should lose you. You must let me talk about it as soon as you can for I want to tell everybody how nice he is. They will know that I should not say so if it was not *very* true. I do not feel ready at this moment to think much about the public good, but I remember, generally, that I did think it would not be a bad thing for you to marry, if you did it well. I shall be looking for your to-morrow's letter, but I feel I know already without telling all that I care most for. What a treasure of a Christmas gift you must feel to have got! It is no use to try to say any more. You will come home soon and let me see that you are still and always will be my old dear Elizabeth. Please give *him* my congratulations. I don't think any one knows better than I do what he will gain.'

Few of Elizabeth's friends rose to these heights. Many were annoyed and uneasy: they expected her to give up her work and it was suggested that for her personal happiness Elizabeth would sacrifice the women's movement. George Eliot's poem, *The Spanish Gipsy*, was quoted. One friend, confident in her worst suspicions, wrote: 'You will not expect me to deny that it is a blow to hear of such a defection.' Voices on the other side were welcome. Prof. Lewis Campbell, who had befriended her in St. Andrews, Mr. Llewelyn Davies and others saw no reason why her professional and public work need suffer by marriage. A man's career did not end with marriage—why should a woman's?

The Rev. Alexander Anderson was somewhat over-whelmed by the 'notoriety' of his future daughter-in-law, but he wrote her a kind, if formal, letter and spelt her surname with an i and one t. In it he gave his son a testimonial: 'James George possesses very superior abilities, an unfailing fund of wit and humour, an equal and most pleasant temper, and his life, as far as known to me, has been pure and honourable.' Annie Peters, the Andersons' old nurse, shared the reverend doctor's doubts about notoriety in a lady. She hoped that 'Miss Garrett was not a scandalous sort of person'—the name of a good woman, she felt, should not appear in print.

At Alde House there was consternation. The attitude of her family towards Elizabeth, usually brimming with approval, was gloomy. Mr. Garrett was crestfallen. He had championed his daughter through thick and thin. With growing pride he had watched her success and now marriage would close her career. Elizabeth realized that her father's attitude was a measure of his pride in her. 'The dear Father gloried in me,' she wrote. To her younger brothers and sisters, sisters especially, she seemed an elderly person. She was thirty-four: Josephine was eighteen. Elizabeth had dedicated herself 'to help wo-men'. She was one of their leaders. That was all very well, but for her to think of marriage was absurd. Who would want to marry her? What could HE be like—a feminist in trousers, probably! It was ridiculous.

Engagement

On Christmas Eve Elizabeth introduced Jamie to her family. He travelled alone but certainly she would meet him at the station. Parents and children waited in the hall where mistletoe and holly decorated the staircase, grandfather clock and ormolu furniture. Newson was gloomy, Agnes and Josephine critical and alert. The wheels of the brougham were heard in the drive. THEY had arrived. A circle of light from the hall fell on the old mare and Lambert in his queer hat. Elizabeth, radiant and self-possessed, appeared first and, then, a tall man. Mrs. Garrett capitulated at once. His courtesy pleased her and he was well versed in doctrinal questions. The manse had seen to that. The young people soon found that they liked him and sent favourable reports to Alice and Millicent, both of whom were married by this time. He was friendly and amusing and spoke with a slight Scottish accent. He proved a great hand at charades, reels, and the Highland Fling for which sometimes he wore a kilt. He sang without accompaniment the *Skye Boat Song, Caller Herrin'* and other national melodies. Josephine suggested *John Anderson, my Jo, John*, and he complied cheerfully. The marshes were frozen. He skated well, indeed, he cut figures on the ice to their admiration. He never mentioned the higher education of women, instead he told them stories. Naturally he won the hearts of Agnes and Josephine, but the puzzle grew. Why should this charming person want to marry Elizabeth? Only Newson remained disappointed and unresponsive.

Engagement

Elizabeth wrote to her sister Millicent:

E.G. to M.G.F.   Aldeburgh, Christmas Day [*1870*]

'I quite meant to write to you yesterday, but on Friday night my horizon was suddenly changed by Mr. Anderson's asking me to marry him. We are engaged. I do hope, my dear, you will not think I have meanly deserted my post. I think it need not prove to be so and I believe that he would regret it as much as I or you would. I am sure that the woman question will never be solved in any complete way so long as marriage is thought to be incompatible with freedom and with an independent career, and I think there is a very good chance that we may be able to do something to discourage this notion.

'He came down one train after me yesterday and is already quite at home with every one. I hope you will like him and that Harry [Professor Fawcett] will too when you meet. This afternoon we have all been on the ice, he introduced himself to Aldebro' on it (having been hidden in the Corporation pew this morning) and won a favourable verdict by beating them all.

'The dear parents are very pleasant about it, tho' the father was I fancy a little disappointed that I should marry at all. However they like him, which is a great point.

'I am very happy, dear Milly. I think we shall be married at Easter—there is nothing to wait for as our joint income will be a very good one and we are both certainly old enough. . . . We have agreed not to be married by the Church of England service and to have no religious service unless we can find one we like. I dare say it will end in our using the Scotch form and bargaining beforehand for no catechism as to obedience. . . .'

The visit to Aldeburgh was short; three days after Christmas Elizabeth was in London, writing her first engagement letter.

E.G. to J.G.S.A.   *London, 28 Dec. 1870*
'Your packet came just in time to send me to bed happy. I had been hungering for a word all day and fresh from our Christmas wealth hunger is hard to bear patiently—at least hard to me who am not patient. I have come to a good many resolutions to-day which you may as well think over before to-morrow night. The first is that I should *very* much like to be married in London, entirely without millinery, and almost without cookery. The second thing I have considered is the duenna [convention demanded a chaperon], and I am clear now that she would be quite a useless plague. My position *must* be accepted as an independent one, and it would be injuring all other professional women a little to allow myself to be treated like a child. When *you* have a duenna I'll have one. Till then we will both be free. It would poison existence to me to have any one near me just now who would take a vulgar or commonplace

Engagement

view of that which is still to me so overpowering and
thrilling. Can you bring some photos of your home
people for me to see? Mr. Anderson and your mother
particularly, I should like to have even a dim image of.
A third resolution relates to money. I should like a common purse to which each contributed and from which
each could draw, better than any elaborate deed of partnership, and division of expenses.'

The engagement lasted six weeks: constant letters
passed between them. Elizabeth's were kept; Jamie's,
with few exceptions, destroyed, as 'no key would keep
them safe'.

E.G. to J.G.S.A.   *11 p.m., 29 Dec. 1870*
'Will you send me back Mrs. Gurney's letter, dearest,
and burn the others? This blessed hour together has *so*
sustained me. I believe my faintness was partly due to
the two days of poor diet. I am not constructed to
flourish on short commons. If you would like to show
your uncle Mrs. Russell Gurney's or any other letter
I send you, I should of course not mind it. It might
comfort him to see that those who know don't think
first of my strong will, etc. I know that that will not be
a rock for us. I am very easy to work with even when
I only respect people, and with *you*—why, the difficulty
will be not to be wickedly facile.'

At an early period of their engagement she had to

169

protect her position as an independent person in a profession.

E.G. to J.G.S.A.   *Undated*
'A Dr. D. who says he is a friend of yours, told some
people that you had told him, "you would not *allow* me
to go on with my practice". Of course I don't believe
it, but it is injurious that he should tell lies about us.
Please stop him.'

Elizabeth usually wrote after her day's work ended;
sometimes in the small hours of the morning. The letters
give an idea of the pressure under which she lived.

E.G. to J.G.S.A.   *London, Wed., 2 a.m.*
'A pile of 50 letters to be read or glanced at has kept
me up, and now I find so much that must be done to-
morrow that I fear even a line would be impossible to
send in the morning. Then at 1 there is St. Mary's [dis-
pensary], at 3.30 a consultation with Andrew Clark, at
4 Miss Davies and after she goes I *must* get down to
Acton to see one of my children [Louie's] who is ailing.
So do not come to-morrow, beloved. Let me have the
Aberdeen brooch. I should like to wear something that
comes from you.'

They discussed plans for the future. He wanted to
provide a smarter house. She thought that for a year or
two they should live in her house, 20 Upper Berkeley
Street, where a smoking-room could be provided, while

Engagement

red curtains and a new tablecloth would beautify the dining-room. He insisted on giving her a carriage and to this she consented. Her professional visits were numerous and great saving of time and fatigue would result. All her tact was needed to persuade him to start married life in her small house.

E.G. to J.G.S.A.   20 Upper Berkeley St., 30 Dec. 1870
'Are you *quite* sure we could not do here for a year or so? I don't want in the least to urge you if you would really dislike it, but I think it is possible that the objection we both felt at first to the idea will wear off as you get used to the house under its new aspect. It would be very foolish to begin too magnificently and a big house does involve a great many other expenses, cut them down as one may. I should so hate you to be worried or to be worried myself about keeping within our income. I do think too, tho' this is of course quite subordinate, that my practice would suffer less if we moved in a year's time, or thereabouts. The two changes, of name and house, will be very trying if taken together. I think too it might be easier to arrange a new house quite satisfactorily when we were more at leisure, and more disposed to spend thought on matters of taste than we are now. We should go to it too with a hoard of probably £1,000 at least saved by not beginning with a heavy outlay. But *please* do not let all this weigh with you if you still think you would feel like a lodger, or

like anything but the head. If we marry in April it must be nearly a year before my name and address would be in the directories and I really think it would be a disadvantage! I should not like to be seriously discouraged by loss of practice in the first year. I think it would be very depressing, and it would make me think I had been the deserter I do not wish or mean to be. If you see any force in these arguments—and mind, I do not *urge* them —I will show you the house on Sunday. I had written all this when your dear ring came. How I rushed down and found only the letter you know without description. But the *only* is very sweet, tho' you do mistake my ambition a little. I am not thinking of myself when I fear the effect you will have on the public side of my life. All that is selfish in me pleads for just *that* that you give me.'

Again:

E.G. to J.G.S.A.　　　　　*London, 31 Dec. 1870*
'The more I think of our future, especially of the first year, the more do I get to hope you would feel it well to come here. I want so much not to fail, in any way, and it would tax me very much either to manage a much larger household well with many patients or to be cheerful in a big house, without them. Besides I should like to be as free as possible from Martha-like cares to take in this great draught of happiness.'

A postscript was added: she suddenly remembered

the date and that when he read her letter the New Year would have started—their New Year of life together. 'Beloved, I shall wish—nay demand—all good things for you from the solemn, veiled Future so close to us. Do so also for me. We *must* grow through this wonderful and thrilling life if we are worthy to receive it and to keep it for ever with us.'

Jamie usually called on Elizabeth in the evening on his way from the city to Hampstead. The joy of being with him overpowered her. She could think of nothing else and this she felt would not do; their meetings should be rationed, she suggested.

E.G. to J.G.S.A.   *2 Jan. 1871*
'I have been sitting half-tranced for nearly an hour since you left me, dearest, and coming to myself I shall ask you not to arrange for us to meet on Wednesday. I am almost sure it will be better for us—for me at any rate, not to meet so very often. It is too distracting. And being very much distracted and absorbed brings back a rush of doubt as to the rightness of taking such absorbing happiness. If you had read *The Spanish Gipsy* you would understand all I mean, and can only so dimly express. But you must not think that the doubts which I admit torment me again and again have the respect of my judgment. They have not; I *know* they are almost morbid, the kind of reaction or revenge inflicted by ambition or by a too exclusive interest in the public side of life.

Engagement

I do not mean to be subdued by them but also I do not want to be continually fighting them. This is why I should like to be married at once, it would put a final end to internal controversy. But as this of course cannot be the next best way of exorcizing the fiend is to keep myself able to attend to other things, to *think* of them. And I can only do this by keeping in some slight degree out of your way. Don't think that in all this there is anything of real hesitation. I am fighting with a nightmare and I know it and yet it teases me.'

These rationed meetings were referred to twenty-four hours later as useful, but she wished him to understand that she intended to have the usual number of letters, which, alas, have been destroyed.

E.G. to J.G.S.A.   20 Upper B. St., 3 Jan. 1871, 10 p.m.
'The starving process is good for working on. I have done more to-day than in any four days before since our Friday, but it's *not* pleasant. I didn't mean to be without a letter, but I dare say that I shall have it for breakfast to-morrow instead. I like to begin the day with a word from you, even when yesterday ended with one, and after 36 hours of fasting to-morrow's dole will be more than ever welcome. I have thought of a delightful little inn to go to when we are married, dear love, if we go anywhere, say from Saturday to Monday. This would not be too great a concession to conventions and perhaps it would be pleasanter not to be in London. The inn is at

the foot of Box Hill near Dorking. If we could succeed in escaping from our friends without any luggage, and if we could without tempting misfortune be married on a Friday, we could have two days' walk over the Leith Hill district, taking our chance for food and resting places. In the winter I should think even walkers would be welcome and if unwelcome your strong presence would get us all we wanted. It would be a great satisfaction to me not to be suspected of being a bride, and no one would I think suspect it, however happy we were, if we were walking and without luggage. We should probably be thought lunatics instead. You see the devil is not tormenting me to-night. I am serenely happy and hopeful. I believe he was strong last night because I had done absolutely nothing but think of you for 48 hours. To-day I have been busy and have had some—not many—brains at the disposal of other people, so that I don't feel that you will be my ruin. I do so wish I could make you at once know all my *memories.*'

This time Jamie's reply was kept, perhaps owing to the criticism it contained. He was a true prophet—'the only possible basis for us is warm personal love and utter truth and out-spokenness'—true also and clear-sighted that he should realize the 'softening influence' their marriage would have on Elizabeth!

J.G.S.A. to E.G.   *Belsize Park, 3 Jan. 1871*
'The only possible basis for us is warm personal love

and utter truth and out-spokenness. Believe me I don't care a button for anything connected with you, but your own self. At the same time it is very pleasant to me that you are a distinguished person. I don't trouble to investigate why that is pleasant—not at present I don't (as the Cockneys say). It is clear to me that I as much dread if not more your dignities as possibly making you vain and unlovely, as I feel pleased and proud of my relation to you their enjoyer. You seem to me very naïve in confessing to ambition. Of course the ideal is to sink one's self and regard only the great principle. If one could only attain to that—recognizably attain to it. What a compelling force! If women are ever to become a power in public matters they must, I think, come nearer visibly than men to this pure ideal. Your confession, my dear love, of "ambition and a too exclusive interest in the public side of life" has reference to that in you which I thought of when I spoke last night of the softening influence of such relations as ours are and I trust will be.'

She welcomed his criticism and had even been looking forward to it.

E.G. to J.G.S.A.   *4 Jan. 1871*
'I have been so happy over last night's dear note, beloved. I was sure before that you would help me up, but I like to feel the process is beginning. I could not love you for ever if you were quite satisfied with me,

being so far from satisfied with myself. Still you do mistake me a little—taking my hesitation as the result of personal ambition instead of what I am sure it is, a dread lest I may be choosing my own happiness at the price of the duty I owe to women who need something which I as one of their leaders can give them.'

Occasionally by happy fortune there was a chance meeting in the city. She passed down Fenchurch Street to get to the Shadwell Hospital. It was better than sunshine if a wave of the hand or a pat on the shoulder gladdened her way to the out-patient department. Sometimes to help chance, directions were given.

E.G. to J.G.S.A.   *6 Jan. 1871*

'I shall look out along Cornhill at 1.45 for the chance of meeting you. My father writes to condole with me on my mother's orthodoxy and her letter, he says, "but it is nothing to what I had, my dear, all the vials were poured on me. I do hope you will do everything that is most proper and usual." How curious it is to see any one of my mother's age so bound in swaddling clothes of formalities! She really wrote as if we were proposing to do something wrong [about their wedding arrangements]. 10 *p.m.* Driving home just now with Dr. Murchison I have tried to comfort him over my defection. He takes my father's line and is very gloomy. You must not make me justify their want of trust. I believe I should almost die of the sense of something akin to guilt, if I

Engagement

found myself, three years hence, really out of the medical field.'

Mr. Garrett's depression about Elizabeth's engagement lingered, but the sight of her happiness and of her continuing medical work helped to disperse it; also he cordially liked his prospective son-in-law.

E.G. to J.G.S.A.   *6 Jan. 1871, 8 p.m.*

'While waiting to be carried off to a consultation I will spend a minute or two with you by way of refreshment. How mud tires one! I have been tramping about in it since 1 this morning, so I have a right to grumble. The carriage will certainly be great economy of fatigue. I heard ourselves discussed to-day in the underground. The narrator wondered what the fellow was like. I had it in my mind to produce your photo. But a glance at the man talking about us forbad that or even any other mode of making myself known to him. He was an enemy tho', which tempted me very much. If he had been a decent sort of looking creature I could not have resisted. I went to Bow from the E.L.C.H. this afternoon as my sister-in-law was ailing. She is very cordial over us, and is quite provoked at the Aldeburgh tone. But then of course she did not glory in me before as the dear father did. Still I am surprised he is still gloomy about it. Have you written at all since we left?'

E.G. to J.G.S.A.   *London, 9 Jan. 1871*

'I hope it will come into your mind to provide a few

178

crumbs for my breakfast to-morrow. How pleasant to have left the region of excuses behind us—in those dim ages before our Friday and to be free to write just because life is intolerable apart! I think you have been very successful to-night with the dear father. He did not say anything in your praise, but he was serene and very affectionate which I understood to be his way of approving. It struck me as quite odd to have his arm round me as we went home in the cab, having now grown so used to yours. His had more of passivity in its affection than your strong grasp has, but when you have had me thirty years and more I shall be very happy, dear love, if there is no more of passivity in yours than now in his. If you starve me to-morrow morning I can't get a word till the evening, as I go to Acton from the E.L.C.H. to see the [Smith] children.'

In addition to her private practice and visits to Shadwell for out-patient work twice a week, Elizabeth had to attend the Guildhall for committees of the School Board and Louie's children expected to see her several times each week. She never failed them but she knew that Jamie would help her to do 'well and wisely' by them and indeed he did.

E.G. to J.G.S.A.   *London, 10 Jan. 1871, 12 p.m.*
'I wonder we missed to-day, for I too was a little late passing along Cornhill at 10′ instead of 15′ to 2. I thought it very hard lines that you should just that once

have been so punctual. I always go by train to Moorgate Street, walk down its east side and along the south side of Cornhill, and I do my best to hit the 1.45 or at latest the 2 train from Fenchurch Street. So we may have better luck next time. At Acton to-night my bairns were disposed to show a great readiness to be cordial to you. They evidently feel it is a momentous change for them, as it is. It is an immense rest to me to feel that we shall be so much more likely to do well and wisely by them than I should have been alone. I made a half promise that we would walk down to see them next Sunday afternoon, if you could manage it. To-night there are 15 letters and I am stupidly tired. Yours, dearest, was the one drop of honey in the budget. Don't think about Portman Square, it is quite out of our reach and would be an endless anxiety. Our reasons for beginning here are quite sound.'

From its extreme formality Mrs. Garrett's note to her future son-in-law sounds less cordial than she intended. It ran:

Mrs. N.G. to J.G.S.A.   *Alde House, 12 Jan. 1871*
'My dear Sir, I received your letter last Monday after-noon with much pleasure, and earnestly hope all your brightest anticipations of happiness will be realized in your marriage with our dear Elizabeth. It is an immense comfort to us both to see that she is so truly happy in her engagement to you, and I cannot but look forward with

more than usual expectations for your mutual happiness and comfort. There are times when the heart is too full to guide the pen—such is the case with me now—I can only commend you both to God's blessing and guidance, truly to know and love Him is life Eternal! Believe me, my dear Sir, sincerely and affectionately yours, Louisa Garrett.'

E.G. to J.G.S.A.   *12 Jan. 1871*

'I am going to settle some accounts to-night and as I find it a fascinating tho' tiresome duty I will spend no more time over pleasure before beginning. It always goes against the grain with me not to finish a thing at a sitting, and happily this requires a long evening with some of my clients. Can you fancy me sending in a bill? I am always a little ashamed of it, and of myself for being so. After our happy hour to-night I have nothing fresh to say, beloved. You will be tired of hearing that which excludes all smaller subjects that I love you more than I thought I was made to love any one.'

The new house was resisted but Jamie was allowed to give Elizabeth a fur jacket as well as a carriage. Referring to the jacket she wrote:

E.G. to J.G.S.A.   *London, 13 Jan. 1871*

'I will get the pattern from the milliner as soon as I have a moment in which to go there. If it would not be ruinous or greedy I should like a not very wide sable border. It is very handsome and it would be a pleasant

variety after the old one. I believe it would be quite safe
to have the sealskin made for a medium-sized woman.
I am exactly what is commonplace, middle size. I have
been docile to-night in the matter of wine, having had
some as a corrective to a long sitting at the Guildhall
and a longer and very cold drive to Wandsworth. Now
it is too late to write anything if Barnett [the maid] is
to spare my going out to the post. I have sent two
photos to Mr. Anderson and have directed the envelope
properly without saying anything about the previous
blunder in my note. "Qui s'excuse s'accuse" strikes me
as a very good proverb. I always avoid excuses as much
as I can and make amends silently.'

Jamie early had to announce that their careers must
be independent of each other.

J.G.S.A. to E.G.   *Undated*
'I think we had better lay it down once for all as a
rule that I am under no circumstances to bring people
"favourably under your notice" or "exert any influence"
or anything of the sort. It will give people a wrong idea
of you unless I take a decided line in this matter—and as
I mean to be if I can a successful man of business neither
interfering with your pursuits nor being interfered with
by you (but having our confidences on all feasible subjects at off times of the day and week and mutually
advising and fortifying one another), I must let people
know unmistakably not to come bothering me about

your public affairs. Will you think about this, dearest?'

Picture galleries gave them both pleasure.

E.G. to J.G.S.A.   *London, 19 Jan. 1871*
'We forgot the Old Masters for Saturday afternoon.
I will be opposite the small Gainsborough blue boy, in
the big room, at 3 and will wait about there ten minutes
or so for the chance of your being able to come. That
happy hour last night quite dispersed the mist—the very
thin one it was—that was trying to come between me
and perfectly serene happiness. In fact it vanished when
you said you had perceived it too! Beloved, we will not
be under the dominion of mists.'

E.G. to J.G.S.A.   *London, 21 Jan. 1871*
'If it would suit you to call here, we could go to the
Old Masters together. I feel sure that I should be shy in
the sealskin unless with you! and it would be pleasant to
consecrate it by five minutes with you before going out
in it. I am beginning to believe that we beat in unison
and harmony, and that when I want you, you want me.
Yesterday's experience did something to convince me
of this, and it had occurred to me before. To-day I have
been wishing in the most weak-minded way for the
middle of March to be quick and come. Fancy, it is only
four weeks to-night since our Friday. It will really make
life seem half as long again as one expected it to be if
time continues for long to move at this snail's pace.

Engagement

After our work was over yesterday Paget[1] gave me his congratulations on my two events. He asked me what I liked best, being the elect of 50,000 or of one. I said I rather despised the 50,000. He thought nothing could be happier on beginning public life than to have 50,000 and to despise them in comparison with one. I liked his quiet way of assuming that I was really beginning public life, not leaving it. I shall be very unhappy if I get no word from you to-night, my dearest. It is true that letters are meagre, after presence, but they are very precious as stop-gaps—like tea and tobacco.'

The revelation of love was overwhelming to Elizabeth, and more so as it came to her in maturity and after a long struggle. During her medical training she had had to face an atmosphere of deep disapproval for years. It was a joy to be free from that. The Job's comforters that now prophesied the worst from her marriage mattered far less. They certainly received only passing attention when they told her that she would sacrifice all she had won, not for herself only, but for women. His friends too pictured him as doomed to oblivion—the husband of a celebrity. How would he like, as the years passed, to have it rubbed into him that the grey mare was the better horse? However the future held great happiness for them both. It is true that theirs was a union of strong wills; but they shared understanding and sympathy, each

---

[1] Sir James Paget, Bart., F.R.C.S.

completing, without hampering, the life of the other.

He, with more imagination, realized the possible stumbling-blocks more clearly than she. They agreed that he was to be master in his own house and not the latest addition to its mistress's furniture. With a sweet and affectionate nature, James George Anderson was a man of character and determination. Elizabeth Garrett's outlook on life was more practical and more religious, but less philosophic, than his. Both, as an axiom, put duty before pleasure. Perhaps she had become slightly arrogant with professional success and with the victory of the School Board election. Her constant proud references to the latter seem to show that this was so. But not for long; his influence softened her and love made her humble and gentle. Arrogance was a veneer, easily removed from the true humility beneath.

E.G. to J.G.S.A.   *London, 22 Jan. 1871*

'Beloved, I have been thinking about those foregone conclusions which you dread and I want to give you some sort of assurance which shall satisfy you. That I love you ought to be enough, and probably is when it presents itself distinctly to you; but in addition to this I can add with complete sincerity that any foregone conclusion which may justify itself to my mind must also be accepted heartily by you before I should let it put itself into practice. It seems to me almost certain that anything which I think—in the light of my love for you

185

—to be right, reasonable, and necessary, will be approved as such by you. I cannot imagine that we should ever take opposed views so long as we both desire to see what is right and reasonable, and to live up to the highest possibilities of our natures. If I thought you incapable of responding to the demands which the common weal makes on every one, and perhaps in some special measure on me, incapable of preferring them if need be, to personal indulgence, you could not be to me what you are. But I am sure I may trust you, and I do trust. You must bear in mind that the daily habit of self-sacrifice is to me as much one of the laws of the highest life as truth is to you. The only foregone conclusion is that we must not be made selfish by love.'

The first of the Married Women's Property Acts had passed in 1869 and Elizabeth felt she should show her approval by taking advantage of its provisions. Jamie, generous to a fault, was a little hurt that she should do so. The Act had not been framed to protect wives from men of his nature.

The marriage took place in the Presbyterian Church, Marylebone, on 9 February 1871. The Rev. James Anderson, D.D., of Morpeth officiated. He was seventy-eight at the time, a magnificent-looking man and known in the family circle as 'the Bishop'. From the first, Jamie had said, 'The Bishop must marry us!' The marriage was 'without millinery' and the bride was not asked to promise obedience, a vow she thought inappropriate and obsolete. At that time marriages had to take place in the forenoon and a 'breakfast' was essential. Professor and Mrs. Fawcett lived on the south side of the Thames and to attend church at 8.30 a.m. would mean an early start. A growler, with straw on the floor, or perhaps a hansom, might bring them and there might be delay at the toll-gate on the bridge.

Shortly before the wedding the bride wrote to urge her sister Millicent to come.

E.G. to M.G.F.   *Undated*

'In all my mass of affairs this week I believe you have never been told the hour [of the service]. It is 8.30. Do come, my dearie, and get Harry up in time too. Breakfast at 0.30.'

8

EARLY YEARS OF MARRIAGE
THE NURSERY

>>➤➡●◄◄◄

Though many campaigns were ahead, Mrs. Anderson's personal difficulties in great measure ended with
marriage. From 1871 to the close of her working life,
some thirty-five years later, she proved that a married woman can succeed in a profession and that a
medical woman need not neglect her family. She built
up her private practice believing that 'to be a great
physician' would help other women more than anything
else she could do, and she devoted herself to public work
mainly on behalf of women in medicine. The prophets
of the engagement period proved to be as false as they
had been gloomy. By marriage she gained in balance
and power and the women's cause was strengthened, not
deserted. 'I did not know I had it in me to care so much
for any one,' is an expression in one of her letters to
Jamie; and to her brother-in-law a week after her
marriage she wrote:

E.G.A. to J. Ford Anderson   *16 Feb. 1871*
'This week has made me know more than I did even

188

Early Years of Marriage—The Nursery

on the 9th [the wedding day] what a prize I have, so you will not wonder if I hold it with a somewhat nervous grasp. It is so much more than I deserve to have such a blessing for all the rest of our lives.'

Great happiness, a perfect partnership, and freedom from worries over petty cash combined to mellow her. She softened. To be laughed at was new to her. No one can remain 'the stern pioneer', at any rate in her own home, if, when she gives herself airs, she is laughed at—and loves it. It was gentle raillery, without a sting, an expression of affection and accompanied by constant and efficient help. Jamie did not understand jealousy, he delighted in his wife's interests, which, to a great extent, he shared. Her position, her success and her achievement pleased him. Her cause became *their* cause.

About the time of Elizabeth's marriage Miss Davies was absorbed in the foundation of Hitchin College, the precursor of Girton. For ten years she had occupied herself with Elizabeth's struggle; it had been her public work, she had been self-effacing and devoted. Now Elizabeth launched in her profession had married the right man. Perhaps Miss Davies thought that, in future, advice and backing might be left to him. At any rate, from this time forwards, she concentrated on Girton and became the first Mistress of the College which was to revolutionize women's education.

For a short time, during 1871, Mr. Anderson was a

member of the executive committee for establishing Hitchin College. However, he did not see eye to eye with Miss Davies over a clause about religious instruction in the memorandum of association and left the committee, to the regret of his wife.

E.G.A. to J.G.S.A.   *16 Nov, 1871*

'At present my impression is that you are making a great deal too much of the points of difference between you and those whom you would call the Conservatives on the committee. It seems to me that women want that which I hope the college will in time give so very very much that those who can help them to it ought not to allow any minor disagreements to take them from the duty of allies. Of course you do not quite share this feeling, to help women is not the passion of your life as it is of mine and Miss Davies. But as in all probability Hitchin (whatever its memorandum may be or its family prayers) will be a hotbed for ultra-Liberalism and as the slight amount of Churchism will probably dispose the young women favourably towards Dissent I think even as a Liberal you ought not to allow such a question to remove you from the list of its supporters.'

Elizabeth and Emily remained friends, but as the years passed they saw less of one another, although Elizabeth remembered with gratitude all that Emily had meant to her 'when in girlhood I sat at her feet'.

From the day Mrs. Anderson returned from a honeymoon almost as brief as Queen Victoria's had been, she was hard at work. Breakfast at 8 a.m. or earlier, if an operation had to be performed, found her with stout boots on and they were not unlaced until the evening. After dinner, piles of letters had to be answered or a speech prepared or lectures written. Occasionally there would be an evening party, attended sometimes with an eye to business, for Lord Granville might be a fellow guest and the chance of discussing the new charter of the University of London must not be lost. However, she liked a party for its own sake: 'I certainly do very much like meeting my fellow creatures, especially when I know them,' and again, 'I begin to think it is one mark of a good heart to like to go to evening parties.' After a day in the city many a husband might have preferred a wife at leisure. Jamie never suggested this. His loyalty was unshakable.

As her practice grew and domesticities increased, it became clear to Mrs. Anderson that efficient work on the London School Board was not possible. She could not give enough time or thought to be a useful member of the board, or to do good work on the sub-committees, and so in 1873 she did not stand for re-election and her place as representative for Marylebone was taken by her sister Alice, Mrs. Herbert Cowell. For a similar reason she resigned the post of honorary assistant physician at the East London Hospital for Children, Shadwell. That she gave this up before another woman had qualified was 'one of the great mistakes of my life', she used to say, and certainly if she had held it longer another medical woman might have been appointed. The next woman elected to the honorary medical staff was Dr. Hazel Chodak Gregory in 1929, more than fifty years later.

During the first seven years of married life, Elizabeth's three children[1] were born and one died. She hated noise and she could not enter readily into a child's mind or play with children; but love overcame these difficulties. She tolerated a baby beating two spoons together as she wrote, and she was a devoted and a wise mother. A nursery makes insistent claims on a mother's time even when the perfect nurse is in charge. Mrs. Anderson was fortunate in finding one in Aaa, who reigned in the nursery of this and the next generation. Aaa's name was Helen Lorimer and she came from Banffshire as a young woman in 1873; saw Mrs. Anderson's children out of the nursery and away to school; then went back to her brother's farm, to return after his death to look after Mrs. Anderson's grandchildren for the rest of her life.

There are few family letters to illustrate these years; probably few were written, as husband and wife seldom separated. Occasionally, however, a new ship building called Mr. Anderson to Glasgow and then of course he was kept in touch with family events.

[1] Louisa Garrett b. July 1873. Margaret Skelton b. September 1874; d. December 1875. Alan Garrett b. March 1877.

Early Years of Marriage—The Nursery

E.G.A. to J.G.S.A.   *London, 18 Feb. 1874*

'There is not much news to tell you. Stacey thinks the
roan is pricked by a nail in the shoe, he has put a poultice
on and sent for the farrier. Alice has been here and thinks
baby looking *very* well indeed and sees her grown during
the last fortnight. I hope the dear *Hesperus* [one of the
firm's last sailing ships] has done her duty well so far
and will not keep you waiting. I am full of sympathy
for the miseries of the passengers. I shall think of you as
coming home on Saturday. Try not to get a bad cold.'

In the spring of the following year it was Mrs. Anderson's turn to leave home. She and her sister Millicent,
the chosen comrade for an expedition, set off to Rome
for a short holiday. A jaunt abroad always filled her with
delight. The nursery appeared serene and was left in the
care of Aaa. They did not leave the beaten track nor
wish to do so. *Baedeker* in hand, the sights were ticked
off until exhaustion called a halt. Foreign speech and
foreign ways provided endless interest; tea was brewed
and consumed in the hotel bedroom from a tumbler—
a great economy and such fun! In some ways she had
a simple mind.

E.G.A. to J.G.S.A.   *On the way to Dover, 18 Mar. 1875*

'So far we are getting on quite well. . . . I wish
you were with me. I shall never elope in real earnest. I
don't like leaving you and the bairns tho' I do most
thoroughly enjoy the sense of holiday—shutting up

books, turning one's mind away from medicine and seeing the out-of-London world. The fields are full of stands of hop-poles now and one is carpeted with very young barley. They are all pretty in the sunlight and seen thro' the wreaths of steam and smoke. I wonder if Louie [aged twenty months] misses me just now at breakfast. Give them daily kisses for me.'

In spite of the joys of Italy it was hard to forget home cares.

E.G.A. to J.G.S.A.   *Florence, 24 Mar. 1875*
'I am grieved to hear of Mrs. Dewar [the wet nurse] and dear wee Margaret having colds. Pray beg nurse to be very careful not to take Margaret out till she has *quite* lost hers. I hope none of their warm wraps have been left off. I shall be anxious to hear again very soon.'

E.G.A. to J.G.S.A.   *Perugia, Good Friday 1875*
'This is the place of all places for our next holyday together, say in September 1876. You would delight in it. I was so very glad that dear baby's cold was going off. . . . Italy is the only place in the world worth busy people spending time upon. We must certainly come here together at our next common outing. I wish so much you were here.'

E.G.A. to J.G.S.A.   *Rome, Mar. 31 1875*
'Your daily letters are very very welcome. It is more than good of you to send them so regularly. . . . I

am longing to see you again. I hope you won't get used
to doing without me. It is very nice to know that Louie
is sweet and nice to you. I meant to have sent her a
picture in this letter but I forgot to get it. Tell her mother
sends her a sweet kiss.'

E.G.A. to J.G.S.A.   *Rome, 2 April 1875*
   'It is very nice to hear of Louie's little advances in
talking and of her being so good and friendly. I wish
Margaret [aged seven months] would be more friendly.
I am longing to see them and you. . . . It seems an
age since I left you.'

   This holiday possessed a special bouquet. The tourists
had an introduction to General Garibaldi and they hoped
to get an audience with His Holiness the Pope, Pio
Nono.

E.G.A. to J.G.S.A.   *Rome, 9 April 1875*
   'I will tell you first about Garibaldi. He lives in a villa
about two miles north of the walls. About half-past two
we reached the villa and were received by Menotti
Garibaldi. He took us at once into the General's room.
Each one was separately introduced and shaken hands
with. He speaks English pretty well. As we were casting
about what to say he asked Menotti if we wanted him
to sign anything and our photos were brought out and
signed. By this time we had recovered a trace of our
self-possession and Milly said to him that Mrs. Seely had

begged to be very kindly remembered to him if we saw him. This led him to talk about the Seelys and as he talked we looked at him. It was one of the most beautiful sights I ever saw, his very fine face, so much finer in expression, in the tenderness of his smile and in clear depth and honesty of his eyes than I had known before, and Millicent's sweet young face and figure expressing any amount of reverence and affection as she looked at him. When he had finished she took one of his stiffened and crippled hands in hers and leant forward (almost I thought as Romola might have done) and said with the sweetest possible grace of tone and manner, "I *think* Mrs. Seely sent her *love* to you." This brought out a very pretty blush on the old man's face and tears into a good many eyes. We tried to get him to say something in support of the women's cause but he did not fully understand our questions and answered somewhat at cross purposes.'

In the summer business took Mr. Anderson to Glasgow.

E.G.A. to J.G.S.A.   *London, 28 Aug. 1875*
'I am sorry you are having a wet journey but if tomorrow is fine it will not much matter. I am just home from a two hours run in the brougham with the children and Aaa. Peeping out of the little window at the back and holding out our hands to catch raindrops have been our chief amusements. Louie [aged two] was much

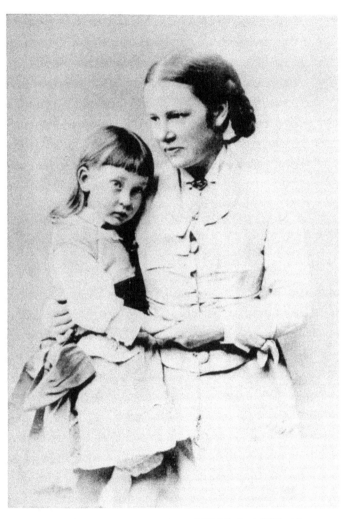

ELIZABETH GARRETT ANDERSON, AGED 40

interested to hear that the rain came straight down from the sky. We saw several patients on the route and ended with the hospital where we saw a wardful all in bed. Louie was delightfully gracious, as if she knew she ought to amuse them and ended by presenting one with a penny she had been nursing in her hand and telling her to buy "chocas" with it. Louie I am sure would send you a kiss but she is upstairs and there is no time to run to her before catching the post.'

Sometimes snatches of holiday together could be fitted in with his visits to Glasgow.

E.G.A. to J.G.S.A.   *London, 21 Sept. 1875*
'I am charmed with the prospect of a week with you in Yorkshire. I have got a guide and a map. I will be at the Station Hotel York by the train that gets there at 7.40 Thursday night. You might have dinner ready for I shall be famished. If it suits you to dine earlier pray do so and let me have some tea and food which would probably suit me better than dinner. The children are *quite* well. We will spend Friday at York, and we can let Nurse know from there where to address us. I am wavering between the dales and the sea but I think it must be the dales. Could you not send home your portmanteau? I shall only bring a bag, so that a pony may carry our baggage. I enjoy the thought of coming so much.'

Early Years of Marriage—The Nursery

That autumn Margaret was ill, but Dr. (later Sir William) Broadbent decided that it was temporary and due to teething. Even so it was worrying, especially with Mr. Anderson in Glasgow, where another ship was on the stocks.

E.G.A. to J.G.S.A.   *London, 4 Oct. 1875*

'We are all as you left us. Baby looks and seems better and has actually walked about 2 yards quite alone. I have had a very busy day and am now proposing to go out with Louie in a hansom for a little fresh air and a rest. I had to make a visit to West Brompton between lunch and the afternoon hospital work which drove me very late there.'

E.G.A. to J.G.S.A.   *London, 5 Oct. 1875*

'We are quite well. Baby looks really like herself to-day and has walked a good many times quite alone. Louie much enjoys walking hand in hand with her. Louie has just been to meet me at the school after Dr. C.'s introductory lecture which has been very good indeed. I feel rather shy of coming after so polished a piece of work. Louie came in afterwards and was introduced. I fancy he can have no children as he did not seem to think as much of her charms as practised judges are wont to do. She was very sweet too and kissed her hand on parting in the most bewitching way.'

Early Years of Marriage—The Nursery

E.G.A. to J.G.S.A.   *London, 7 Oct. 1875*

'I am very sorry not to have written before but I have not had a moment of spare time, or rather the moments I had set aside for you were seized upon unexpectedly. Louie has looked rather peeky all day and has eaten badly. She went into a passion of anger and annoyance just now because I ate a morsel of her "bucker" half in fun and half for my hunger as I had missed my own bucker and was sick and tired. Till then however she had been sweet and nice to me. I have been busy this week and am therefore well and in good spirits. I hope you are so too, dearest. I was sorry not to hear from you this morning.'

The ailing baby gave more anxiety and convulsions occurred.

E.G.A. to J.G.S.A.   *London, 9 Oct. 1875*

'We have had a sad fright over dear baby. She is better now but she has been much more ill than ever before, last night she had a convulsion. It was not severe nor very long and in less than twenty minutes she was fully conscious again. This morning she is drowsy and languid. She is *quite* conscious when awake, notices Louie, asks for her doll. Ford [Dr. J. Ford Anderson] seemed to fear this morning that there might be some brain mischief but Dr. Broadbent agrees with me in thinking the evidence is entirely against this and that it is simply reflex irritation from the teeth. He still assured me you need not be alarmed. This is his opinion this morning as well as last night and in spite of her still being evidently in distress.'

E.G.A. to J.G.S.A.　　　　　　*London, 11 Oct. 1875*

'I don't know what to say about baby. There are no more signs of convulsions, but the fever keeps up. The night was evidently very restless. Nurse did not come for me and as I had Louie and was late in settling I did not go up till about 7. When Dr. Broadbent came I urged his lancing the left side gums again and he did so. She has been more comfortable and able to sleep since. I do not see any signs of serious illness, i.e. threatening life and I quite anticipate her being very much better in a few days. Still she is now very ill, poor pet, and my chief reason for half asking you to come home was feeling that it was possible I might knock up before she was quite well. I don't think I shall but if I did I would like you to be here to look after her. It is hard work physically carrying her about and pacing the room hour after hour and it is not impossible that it might put me for a time *hors de combat*. I am not going out and am seeing scarcely any one even here. With getting Nurse some rest in the day and all the little ministerings to baby there is quite enough to do.'

Margaret grew worse. She developed tubercular peritonitis and died in December 1875 at the age of fifteen months. Towards the end, mother and nurse, quite exhausted, had to rest. Jamie took their place, and with the dying child on his shoulder, paced up and down the nursery floor—patting her as he walked—heavy, gentle, firm pats. The cries ceased. Her pain was eased but, if he rested, she whimpered. Would the night ever end? A streak of light told of the dawn. A dog barked outside: Margaret raised her head against her father's cheek: 'Bow-Bow,' she said and then peace came.

E.G.A. to M.G.F.   *Undated (Dec. 1875)*

'Thank you so much for your tender loving sympathy. It *is* a hard blow. We laid the dear child in her little grave yesterday. . . . Louie came home with us and we have begun life again on its altered scale and in a tender key—but I am sure we both feel very thankful to have had even one year of the dear little life with us. Louie is of course half puzzled and half unconscious. She says pretty often "Babee now—ta ta Babee!" which is hard to hear composedly.'

The parents were heartbroken and they did not understand the source of the trouble. That tubercle bacilli could be carried by milk was not realized at that time. Margaret had been 'given the milk from one cow', according to regulation. It had been an infected, untested cow and she had died from repeated doses. Her mother thought the tubercle must be hereditary and that other children of hers might develop the same trouble. Two years later Alan was born and Mrs. Anderson tried to steel herself against loving the new baby over-much. It would hurt her less, if he had to die, that he should not engross her heart. No doubt he dealt with the situation promptly.

The next batch of family letters were written when Alan was two years old (1879) and Mr. Anderson was in Scotland at the shipyards again, this time supervising a steamer.

E.G.A. to J.G.S.A.   *London, 5 June 1879*

'Baby [Alan] is still not quite well. He had a restless night and took no breakfast. Tongue white and skin hot. No cough, and not too ill to play with Louie thro' my breakfast. I did not let him go out, and he has had a good sleep this forenoon, is now *extremely* merry just at his jolliest and quite cool. So I think the heat must be due to toothache and that we need not be anxious. However I shall not go to Aldeburgh this week, and will keep a careful watch over him. He sends you 200 kisses and Louie sends 2,000 million. She is full of life and *quite* well. She says she can't help being a little glad I am not going to Aldeburgh tho' she knows I would like to go. She is a particularly considerate creature, tho' she knows very well what she likes for herself.'

E.G.A. to J.G.S.A.   *London, 14 Oct. 1879*

'We are all quite well. Louie was delighted with your long letter. Alan [aged two and a half] very pertinently remarked after hearing it read, "When Papa come home? Baby likes Papa." I am very glad you had such a good day amongst the hills on Sunday. We were burning candles and gas all the forenoon. I am pegging away very comfortably at my lectures—not very busy in other ways. The children and I are all enjoying our little times [she read to them from six to seven every evening] very much. The winter has many merits to make up for fog and cold. You might bring or send Louie some little pictures of the Lake country to excite her desire to see it.'

Mrs. Anderson enjoyed good music and went to concerts as often as possible. She helped to found a Home Quartet Society, the members of which held musical evenings at their houses by turn.

E.G.A. to J.G.S.A.   *London, 25 Oct. 1881*
'I was so sorry when I returned last night and found you gone. It has been a chapter of accidents altogether. The attraction of the evening was Beethoven's splendid choral symphony and this by a most perverse arrangement was put at the end of the concert. Till 10 o'clock there was dreary music which bored me very much. I have just had a long visit from Mr. Trelawny's niece (my patient). She came back from Rome last night, after getting the poor old fellow cremated at Gotha and the ashes placed by the side of Shelley's in the tomb at Rome. His daughter refused to carry out his will in these particulars, so the niece who is one of the timid brave

women with nerves of a mouse and heart of a lion did it all herself. At the Italian frontier she was so afraid the precious ashes would get spilt by the rough ways at the Custom House that she rolled the canister up in her shawl and kept it under her arm. This was looked upon in Rome as smuggling to evade the customs dues and the poor soul was kept there six weeks before she could get leave to bury her canister in the right place. We are all quite well. Bay [Alan] has just been for a good ride. I hope you will take real good care of yourself and try not to catch cold.'

Col, the collie dog 'with a brow like Shakespeare's', was an important member of the household and a constant companion to the children.

E.G.A. to J.G.S.A.   *London, 21 May 1882*
'Coming back by Metropolitan Railway [from a family call] we had a very innocent-looking German gentleman in the carriage with us who seemed to admire Col greatly. Col in turn was attracted by him. Sitting opposite, Louie in a loud whisper said, "Mardle, don't you think he *may* be a dog-stealer? *Are* his boots big enough to hold a bit of meat?" Presently coming upstairs Col would get in front, took a wrong turn and was not to be seen when we were in the street. Louie and Bay were convinced the man *was* a dog-stealer. However Aaa found Col on the City side peering into

all the carriages for us and of course we received the
truant with enthusiastic affection.'

During another Italian holiday Mrs. Anderson had to
return suddenly. Alan had developed measles. She wrote
to her husband from Venice. 'If I hear from you that
you will positively be at Dover I will come to you at
the Lord Warden and this would keep you in bed and
prevent your night from being spoiled. But you must
manage so that it looks quite proper and also that I don't
get turned into the wrong person's bedroom.'

In these years of early marriage Mrs. Garrett Anderson
proved that a medical woman can do her duty as a wife
and mother and that a wife and mother need not forfeit
medical practice. While she was fully occupied with her
profession, with the cares of a young family and the
heart-break of losing a child, Miss Jex-Blake took the
lead in founding the London School of Medicine for
Women. It was a great achievement, and through the
school the ordered progress of women in medicine
became possible.

9

THE LONDON SCHOOL
OF MEDICINE FOR WOMEN

>>➤➤●◄◄◄

Until 1869 Elizabeth Blackwell and Elizabeth Garrett
were the only women practising medicine in England,
and the doors by which they had entered the profession
had been closed to other women. In March of that year
an important event occurred. Recruits appeared. First,
Sophia Jex-Blake applied to the University of Edinbrugh
for medical training, and soon afterwards six other
women joined her. To their surprise and joy the University allowed them to matriculate in the Faculty of
Medicine. Their lectures and demonstrations were taken
apart from the other students, their fees being propor-
tionately increased, and they settled down to hard and
happy work. For some years Miss Garrett and Miss Jex-
Blake had known each other. During Elizabeth's student
days both had been members of the Rev. F. D. Maurice's
congregation, they had belonged to the same debating
society and they had friends in common, in particular
Elizabeth's much-loved sister Louie. At one time Sophia
Jex-Blake was teacher of mathematics at Queen's Col-

lege; then she went to America, where contact with women physicians led her to adopt medicine as her career.

Miss Garrett and Miss Jex-Blake did not suit each other, but they had the same aim—to help other women to wider opportunities—and Miss Garrett was delighted to hear of the venture in Edinburgh and to have colleagues in the making. She interested Lady Amberley in the women students.

Lady Amberley's Diary   *14 Aug. 1869*
'Miss Garrett is anxious to get some scholarships at Edinburgh for the women who are likely to be allowed to study there as medical students next winter as the senate have admitted them and it has only to be confirmed by the General Council and Chancellor. I have settled to give one of the scholarships of £50 for three years. Miss Garrett gives a third of another.'

Miss Garrett welcomed the advent of the women students in Edinburgh but she found that co-operation with Miss Jex-Blake was not easy. Miss Jex-Blake looked upon her as a brilliant individual and an asset to the general movement. No one, however, could follow in her footsteps as the Society of Apothecaries had altered its charter in order to exclude women. Miss Garrett's obvious duty was to pursue her practice diligently and to show the world that a woman could be a reliable physician. Miss Jex-Blake felt that she had dropped the cause as a whole, and that a fresh pioneer effort was needed if women were to be admitted to the profession. She determined to open another door and among the women in Edinburgh she was the acknowledged leader.

They worked as only pioneers will and their success in the class examinations was conspicuous. The majority took honours, and Miss Edith Pechey won, or should have won, the Hope Scholarship for Chemistry, a coveted honour in the University. The Professor of Chemistry refused to award it to a woman, and so it went to the man below her on the examination list. The storm now broke. On the side of the women there rose the cry of injustice, and sympathy with them was widespread and influential. The University Court, with the concurrence of every other body in the University, had accepted the women as matriculated students. The professors in the Faculty of Medicine now defied the Court, refused to teach them and acquiesced in, if they did not stimulate, the hostility of a section of the students. Sir Robert Christison led the official opposition and being a member of every important body whose decision counted—the Medical Faculty, the Senatus, the University Court, the University Council and the Infirmary Board—he carried great weight. His hostility was intense. In the so-called 'Riot of Surgeons' Hall', when mud and filth were thrown, Miss Jex-Blake was told that Professor Christison's assistant led the students. She repeated this at a public meeting, and a libel action was brought against her. The law pursued its slow and expensive course. Proceedings lasted two years, the result being that the plaintiff was awarded one farthing; while costs, amounting to £1,000, were assessed against the defender. A committee to promote the medical education of women in Edinburgh was formed (November 1871) with Miss Louisa Stevenson—a connection by marriage of Mr. J. G. S. Anderson—as the honorary secretary. It included over five hundred members who supplied valuable moral support and defrayed the costs in the Christison action and other legal expenses which followed.

Some of the principal men in Edinburgh supported the women students. Professor Masson championed them, and the friendship of the Lord Provost (Mr. Alexander Russell) and of the Editor of the *Scotsman* (Mr. William Law) was invaluable. Feeling in Edinburgh ran high. A hostess had to choose her company with care. Even a good dinner would not bridge the gulf between the 'ayes' and the 'noes' over the women's question. Litigation, in which the women students were parties, continued from 1871 for three years. In 1873 by the advice of the Lord Advocate, Miss Jex-Blake brought an action against the Senatus praying to have it declared that the University was bound to enable the women students to finish their education and to sit for a qualifying degree. The women won this action, but next year on appeal to the Court of Session, the verdict was

The London School of Medicine for Women

reversed by a majority of one—'the University had exceeded its powers when it admitted women to matriculate.' Defeat was completed by the refusal of the Board of the Infirmary to admit women to clinical instruction.

Miss Jex-Blake might have carried the appeal to the House of Lords but funds were exhausted. For the present she decided to withdraw from Edinburgh and to make a fresh effort elsewhere. She and Mrs. Isabel Thorne, one of her fellow students, came to London. Some of the others went to Zürich and Paris.

From this time forward Mrs. Anderson and Miss Jex-Blake inevitably saw a good deal of one another. They were cast in different moulds; friendship was out of the question, co-operation uneasy. Mrs. Thorne, who respected and liked them both, acted as intermediary. Dr. Margaret Todd[1] says: 'Mrs. Anderson looked through the wrong end of the telescope at Sophia Jex-Blake.' Perhaps she did. At any rate they paid one another the compliment of outspoken sincerity. Up to this time the pioneers had avoided public disagreement. Now, on the issue 'expatriation' or 'fight it out on this line' (S.J.-B.'s expression), they proclaimed their differences. How were women to reach the Medical Register? Foreign education and a foreign diploma had no legal value in England. As Miss Jex-Blake wrote, 'few things would please our opponents better than to see one Englishwoman after another driven out of her own country to obtain medical

[1] *Life of Sophia Jex-Blake, M.D.*

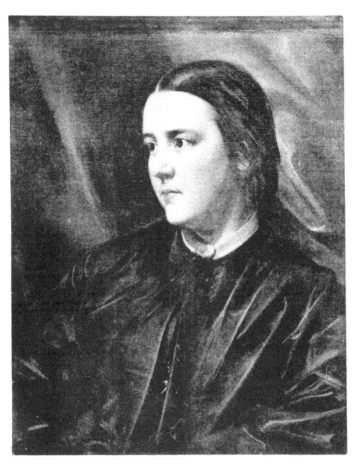

SOPHIA JEX-BLAKE, AGED 25
from the portrait by Samuel Lawrence

education abroad because they know that on her return after years of labour she can claim no legal recognition whatever.' She determined to find a way in which women could enter the medical profession in compliance with English law.

The Medical Act 1858 governed the situation. Passed before the appearance of medical women for the protection of the public against quacks, it enacted that no medical practitioner could register unless he held a licence, diploma or degree granted by a British examining body, and all nineteen examining bodies refused to accept women candidates. Mrs. Garrett Anderson was inclined to minimize this objection and expressed her views in *The Times*.

E.G.A. '*The Times*'   *5 Aug. 1873*
'. . . The real solution of the difficulty will, I believe, be found in Englishwomen seeking abroad that which is at present denied to them in their own country. . . . By going to Paris female students can get without further difficulty or contention, at a very small cost, a choice of all the best hospital teachers of the place, a succession of stimulating and searching examinations, and a diploma of recognized value. The one serious drawback to the plan is, that the Paris degree, in spite of its acknowledged worth, does not entitle its holder to registration as a medical practitioner in this country. . . . "Nothing succeeds like success," and if we could

The London School of Medicine for Women

point to a considerable number of medical women quiety making for themselves the reputation of being trustworthy and valuable members of the profession, the various forms which present opposition now takes would insensibly disappear, and arrangements would be made for providing female medical students with the advantages which it appears hopeless to look for at present in this country.'

Miss Jex-Blake disagreed entirely with Mrs. Anderson's suggestions. She replied on August 23rd[1] and began by saying she had 'only just seen Mrs. Anderson's letter'.

S.J.-B. 'The Times'   23 Aug. 1873·

'. . . I venture to beg that you will allow me to point out my reasons for thinking she [Mrs. Anderson] has selected the very worst of all the alternatives suggested when she advises Englishwomen to go abroad for medical education. . . .' Argument followed: she continued, '. . . I trust therefore that I have shown that Mrs. Anderson's advice . . . is premature in the extreme. I hope further to show that it is moreover radically erroneous in principle. . . . Let me . . . conclude . . . by protesting as strongly as lies in my power against this idea of sending abroad every Englishwoman who wishes to study

[1] This letter, dated 8 Aug., appears in *Life of Sophia Jex-Blake* by Dr. Margaret Todd, but reference to the files of *The Times* gives the later date, 23 August.

medicine; let me entreat all such women to join the class already formed in Edinburgh, the great majority of whose members are thoroughly of one mind with me in this matter and who, having counted the cost, are like myself, thoroughly resolved to "fight it out on this line" and neither to be driven out of our own country for education nor to be induced to cease to make every effort in our power to obtain from the Legislature that measure of justice which we imperatively need, and which is, in point of fact, substantially implied in the provisions of the Medical Act of 1858.'

By 1874 Miss Jex-Blake's plans were mature and she told Mrs. Anderson what she meant to do. She proposed *at once* to found a separate medical school for women in London. She thought that a general hospital would be found willing to provide clinical instruction for the students and that the examining boards would recognize a 'properly equipped medical school'. This seemed high optimism. The plans were 'almost completed', she told Mrs. Anderson, and 'leading medical men had consented to join the teaching staff'. She felt 'almost confident of the ultimate success of the School'. Acting with characteristic energy she came from Perthshire to London and saw Dr. Anstie, Hon. Physician to King's College Hospital, and Mr. Norton, Hon. Surgeon to St. Mary's Hospital. Both were encouraging and approved her scheme. They had been in Edinburgh during the struggle and had become her warm friends. She did not ask Mrs. Anderson's advice, but she formed a provisional council for the proposed new medical school and asked her to join it not only 'in order to avoid any public suggestion of a split in the ranks' but 'for her future reputation'. This opening made it difficult for Mrs. Anderson to co-operate. Her opinion was entitled to consideration as the failure of the attempt would have damaged the cause immeasurably. Mrs. Anderson had been in practice for nine years and had won her way against prejudice and hostility to a position of consideration and influence, both socially and in the profession. Miss Jex-Blake had led a gallant struggle in Edinburgh, but she had failed and she was unqualified and without any prospect of qualifying. No one knew better than Mrs. Anderson how great the odds were against success, and she realized that to make the attempt and to fail would be disastrous. Miss Jex-Blake's impetuous way of rushing ahead and ignoring difficulties was not re-assuring. To start a school was a most serious undertaking. The labour involved would be prodigious. Mrs. Anderson thought the time was 'not ripe'. For herself at the moment she wanted no more responsibilities and the personality of the prospective founder made her hesitate. Her letter to Miss Jex-Blake has been lost, but a copy of the reply was preserved.

S.J.-B. to E.G.A.   *Hampstead, 21 Aug. 1874*
'If I kept a record of all the people who bring me

cock-and-bull stories about you, and assure me that you are "greatly injuring the cause", I might fill as many pages with quotations as you have patience to read. . . . Nor do I much care to know whether or no certain anonymous individuals have confided in you that they lay at my door what you call "the failure at Edinburgh". . . . It can, as I say, serve no purpose whatever to go into this sort of gossip . . . but, quite apart from any such discussion, I am more than willing to say that if, in the opinion of a majority of those who are organizing this new school, my name appears likely to injure its chances of success, I will cheerfully stand aside, and let Mrs. Thorne and Miss Pechey carry out the almost completed plans. So much for your second objection (to joining the Council of the School) which I have taken first. . . . In conclusion let me say that I never said it "did not signify" whether you joined the Council (though I did say that I believed the School was already tolerably certain of ultimate success). I think it is of very great importance, both for your credit and ours, that there should, as you say, be no appearance of split in the camp, and I should greatly prefer that your name should appear on the council with Dr. Blackwell's and those of the medical men who are helping us.'[1]

Mrs. Garrett Anderson joined the council and served the school to the end of her life.

[1] Reprinted from *Life of Sophia Jex-Blake* by Dr. Margaret Todd.

The London School of Medicine for Women

During the weeks that followed, Miss Jex-Blake kept in close touch with Mr. A. T. Norton and Dr. Anstie. Mr. Norton was convinced that 'a thoroughly good medical school might be organized apart from the existing schools', the staff being composed of teachers from other schools recognized by the examining bodies. Dr. Anstie was young and brilliant. His position in the profession was high and he had many friends. It was a stroke of fortune to enlist the help of such a man. His indignation had been roused by the treatment of the women in Edinburgh and he said to Miss Jex-Blake, 'I wonder that the public do not rise against the medical profession and stone us with paving stones.' He became an ardent supporter of the cause of medical women. The temporary office of the London School of Medicine for Women (name given by the founder) was in his house, 69 Wimpole Street. With the help of advisers such as he, Miss Jex-Blake collected a provisional council which first met at his house, 22 August 1874. Those present were Dr. Anstie, Miss Sophia Jex-Blake, Miss Edith Pechey, Mr. Norton, Dr. Burdon Sanderson, Dr. Buchanan, Mr. Critchett, Dr. Cheadle, Dr. Sturgis and Mrs. Garrett Anderson. Dr. Anstie was elected dean of the school. Miss Jex-Blake was the ruling spirit, and, by her own wish, only registered medical practitioners were invited to form the provisional council. It was a self-denying ordinance but no doubt she looked forward to a day, not far distant, when she would be qualified to join the

The London School of Medicine for Women

council, and control the school, for it was her child. An official honorary secretary was not appointed, secretarial work and organization being left to Miss Jex-Blake, although her name did not appear on the prospectus. She worked like a hero. Lecturers were appointed and, with the exception of Mrs. Garrett Anderson, they were teachers in other medical schools, recognized by the Colleges of Physicians and Surgeons. The staff was chosen carefully, not merely as first-rate teachers, but in order that they might plead effectually, each in his own circle, for the recognition of the new school.

Surely, after such precautions, the object of the promoters—to persuade the licensing bodies to recognize the school as able to instruct students for qualifying examinations—would be gained? At any rate it could not be turned down on the ground of an inferior professional staff. Dr. Anstie wrote to the Apothecaries' Company, to the Secretary of the Royal College of Surgeons of London, and to the Registrar of the Royal College of Physicians of England. Their refusals followed but meanwhile the campaign continued. Miss Jex-Blake and Mrs. Thorne found thirteen contributors who each gave one hundred pounds, and the lease of 30 Henrietta Street, its furniture and equipment were bought with this sum. 'Actually signed lease and got possession of 30 Henrietta Street,' is the triumphant entry in Miss Jex-Blake's diary 15 September 1874.

The slender resources of the council were exhausted

over these initial expenses. They had a small purse for their great undertaking but a calamity worse than an empty exchequer now overtook them. As the preliminary arrangements were completed Dr. Anstie died of blood poisoning on 12 September. It was tragic. Of all the people connected with the school at that time, he seemed the most vital and important. To fill his place, Mr. A. T. Norton agreed to become dean—a post he held for nine years, with much advantage to the school. On 12 October the London School of Medicine for Women opened. Of the fourteen original students, twelve had been working in Edinburgh. The newcomers were Miss Fanny Butler, later a medical missionary in Kashmir, in whose memory a scholarship has been founded, and Miss Jane Waterston, who became a public person of importance in South Africa, and who at her death fifty years later bequeathed a legacy to her old medical school.

Mr. Norton did not let the grass grow under his feet. On the day following the opening he wrote to fourteen examining bodies to ask them to place the school on their lists of recognized medical schools. In due course refusals came from them all. A few days later he turned his attention to the second imperative need of the school —a general hospital, in the wards of which the students could receive clinical training. Mrs. Garrett Anderson hoped that the London Hospital, which had not many students, might consent, but negotiations broke down owing to opposition from some members of the medical staff. The Royal Free Hospital in Gray's Inn Road possessed sufficient beds to meet legal requirements and no medical school was attached to it. Surely its prestige would go up if it became a teaching hospital? Why should the women students not be welcomed in its wards? Mr. Norton wrote in his most persuasive manner but the reply was a curt refusal.

In May 1875 the provisional council handed over the school to a body of governors, consisting of themselves and others, including the Earl of Shaftesbury, Professor Huxley, the Dowager Lady Stanley of Alderley, and many more. A smaller executive council was to be elected annually from the governing body, and at its third meeting, Mrs. Garrett Anderson was appointed one of the lecturers in medicine. Funds did not permit of the simultaneous delivery of lectures on every subject but by a rotation of classes the whole curriculum would be covered in three years. The classes for the second year, when five new students were admitted, were anatomy, practical anatomy, physiology, surgery, medicine, midwifery, forensic medicine and ophthalmic surgery.

The veteran Lord Shaftesbury presented the prizes at the first and second winter sessions. His life had been spent in one humanitarian effort after another. Lunatics, climbing boys [chimney-sweeps], women and children in mines and factories and many others had occasion to bless his name. Now, as an old man, he extended his help and earned gratitude from the women struggling to qualify in medicine. His presence, however, was not enough to solve the difficulties of the new school. More students joined, but its prospects were exceedingly gloomy. With no hospital to teach the students and no examining body to examine them, it seemed as if it must close. The minutes of the executive council, February 1876, reflect these anxieties: 'Several students have left owing to the inability of the school to provide qualifying hospital practice. They have reason to fear a still further decrease in numbers from the same cause.' And again: 'The Executive Council feel the utmost regret in stating that they have been unable to make arrangements with any of the existing hospitals for a qualifying course of hospital attendance for the students of the school and they cannot conceal their conviction that this point is of such capital importance that on it must eventually turn the very existence of the school.' Public attention was called to the situation. The Government, through the Lord President of the Privy Council, applied to the General Medical Council for their opinion on the subject of the admission of women to the medical profession. In reply the General Medical Council reported that such admission presented 'special difficulties', but that 'the Council are not prepared to say that women ought to be excluded from the profession'. Legislation was required.

The London School of Medicine for Women

In March a deputation from the school consisting of Lord Aberdare, Mrs. Garrett Anderson, Miss Jex-Blake, Dr. King Chambers, Mr. Norton and the Rt. Hon. James Stansfeld, M.P., waited upon the Duke of Richmond and Gordon, Lord President of the Privy Council, to urge Government intervention.

Speaking on the deputation, Mrs. Garrett Anderson explained that a two-fold difficulty lay in the way of the admission of women to the Register. The only body that did not profess to be able to exclude women as women was the Society of Apothecaries and they practically refused them admission, inasmuch as they would only examine those who were educated at the public medical schools already recognized, and from these schools women were excluded. It was true that on the continent women could obtain an excellent education in medicine but then no foreign diploma was now admitted to registration in this country. The complete school of medicine organized for women was not recognized by the examining boards, and its students were refused admission at all metropolitan hospitals. It was pointed out that special privileges were not desired but merely the removal of special disabilities.

No immediate success followed and the fortunes of the school were low. It was clear that the school must close after the next winter session unless clinical teaching could be obtained for the students. At this darkest hour, light came. Victory was won.

The London School of Medicine for Women

The Rt. Hon. Russell Gurney, M.P., introduced a short permissive bill giving all British medical examining boards the right to admit women to their examinations. This became law on 12 August 1876 as the Medical Act 1876. The walls of the fort crumbled. Mr. Russell Gurney was triumphant.

Rt. Hon. R.G. to S.J.-B.   *London, 21 July 1876*
'I saw Lord Shaftesbury yesterday and he intends to give notice on Monday to move the second reading on Tuesday. The third reading will probably follow in a day or two. All that we shall then have to wait for will be the Royal Assent.'

After this important event, the executive council framed its report to the governing body in a very different tone. Special thanks were tendered to Lord Aberdare and Lord Shaftesbury, also to the Rt. Hon. W. Cowper Temple, the Rt. Hon. Russell Gurney, the Rt. Hon. John Bright and Dr. Cameron, to whose efforts this result was mainly due.

Miss Edith Pechey and Miss Edith Shove went to Ireland and won the consent of the King and Queen's College of Physicians, now the Royal College of Physicians, Ireland, to take advantage of the recent permissive legislation to recognize the London School of Medicine for Women and to admit its students to their examinations. 'Miss Pechey has done wonders,' wrote Mrs. Isabel Thorne. The London School was inspected

and placed on the list of recognized medical schools—
thus at last women obtained a registrable licence.

In the forefront of Miss Jex-Blake's services to medical women stands the introduction of the Rt. Hon.
James (later Sir James) Stansfeld to the school. In 1871,
during a visit to London from Edinburgh, she met him.
He was an intimate friend of Professor and Mrs. Masson
who, at that time, were much moved by the struggle of
the women students in Edinburgh. Miss Jex-Blake impressed him and he introduced her to some of his colleagues in the Cabinet. When later she urged him to
become honorary treasurer of the fledgeling medical
school, he agreed. Early in 1877 he, as honorary treasurer, was deputed to try to negotiate arrangements for
clinical teaching in the Royal Free Hospital. The friendly
attitude of the chairman of the general committee, Mr.
James Hopgood, who no doubt was influenced by Mrs.
Hopgood, a supporter of the women's movement,
helped greatly.

Rt. Hon. J.S., M.P. to S.J.-B.   *Undated, 1876*

'I met Mrs. Garrett Anderson at dinner the other day.
She did not seem to have much hope or plan about the
School in any way. I have however something to tell
you that I think you will be rather pleased to hear.
Mrs. Stansfeld and I went to Clapham to-day to call
on the Hopgoods, with whom we had become friendly
at Whitby and Mr. Hopgood is Chairman of the Board

The London School of Medicine for Women

of the Gray's Inn Lane [Royal Free] Hospital. We found them both with us but strange to the question. I am to send Mr. Hopgood something to read and he is to consider whether anything is possible there—*he does not appear to be in awe of the staff.* . . . In dealing with Mr. Hopgood I very much wish you were here. What time in January shall you be back, probably time enough for us to act together in the matter.' [From *Life of Sophia Jex-Blake*.]

Apparently for once things went more easily than had been expected. Mr. Stansfeld and Miss Jex-Blake visited Mr. Hopgood. Later the happy news was sent by telegram.

Rt. Hon. J.S. to Miss S.J.-B. Telegram, 15 Mar. 1875
'Royal Free Hospital have unanimously accepted my proposal. Come before 10 o'clock Saturday. I go out half past ten. Stansfeld.'

A tentative five years' agreement was concluded between the hospital and the school. In return for clinical teaching of their students, the school undertook to pay the hospital an annual sum of £715.[1] Five hundred guineas were to go to the medical staff and the balance towards the general expenses of the hospital. Three friends gave their personal guarantee to the hospital for this money, the exchequer of the school being empty:

[1] The hospital remitted this payment when the second agreement was signed.

they were Mr. Stansfeld, M.P., Mr. Frederick Pennington, M.P., and Mr. J. G. S. Anderson.

The executive council of the school reported in May: 'Mainly by negotiations between Mr. Stansfeld and Mr. Hopgood, Chairman Royal Free Hospital, an agreement has been negotiated for the clinical work of women students.'

In these efforts Mrs. Garrett Anderson did not take an active part. Five days before the glad news reached her that the Royal Free Hospital had opened its wards to women students, she brought into the world the son who half a century later was to become its chairman.

During the first three experimental years of the school, thirty-four students had entered and their fees amounted to £1,249 10s. In addition, two thousand pounds had been subscribed by friends privately. A public meeting to launch an appeal for funds was held at St. George's Hall in June 1877. Lord Shaftesbury, K.G., presided. Professor Henry Fawcett moved the resolution 'that this meeting regards with the greatest satisfaction the progress of the movement for promoting the education of women in medicine and their admission to the ranks of the medical profession.' At the present moment, he said, all that was needed was money—simply money. The appeal for £5,000 was successful, £3,464 being raised at the meeting and £5,255 being reached shortly afterwards. At about the same time the school received its first important bequest from the will of Mrs. George Oakes of Parramatta, New South Wales.

This year chronicled another advance. Twelve months earlier a distinguished student of the school, Miss Edith Shove, had applied to the University of London for admission to examination in the Faculty of Medicine. The Senate agreed, but Convocation protested against the admission of women to medical degrees before the question of their admission to all degrees had been settled. The Senate then prepared a supplementary charter providing that all degrees should be open to women. During the discussion in convocation on the draft charter, Sir William Jenner, K.C.B., M.D., said 'he had one dear daughter and he would rather follow her to the grave than see her subjected to such questions as could not be omitted from a proper examination for a surgical degree.' It is said that raising both his hands he prayed that those 'who knew but little on this subject might follow those who ought to know a great deal about it'. (*Standard*, 16 January 1878.) That Miss Jenner in later life became an ardent feminist and worked for the parliamentary enfranchisement of women may have been a reaction from her upbringing.

In spite of such opposition the result of the voting was: Ayes 242; Noes 132. The charter was approved and medical women could at last obtain a degree through all the successive stages open to men.

While the charter was under consideration, Lord

The London School of Medicine for Women

Granville called on Mrs. Garrett Anderson. He was famed for courtesy, but at the end of their interview his attitude was uncertain. At that moment, from behind a sofa, the daughter of the house, aged four, appeared. Up till then she had played no part in the interview; now, with a doll in her arms, she told the Chancellor, 'You may kiss him.' To the parents this incident seemed decisive.

The events of 1877 launched the school. A new era opened before it. But, to the founder, came a blow which changed her plans and, perhaps, her life. Up till this time, Dr. Sophia Jex-Blake had done the secretarial work for the school and most of the organization; now it was decided to appoint an official honorary secretary. At a meeting of the council the names of Dr. Jex-Blake and Mrs. Garrett Anderson were considered for this post. Dr. Jex-Blake was not present and Mrs. Garrett Anderson suggested that the election should be postponed. At the following meeting, Mrs. Isabel Thorne, who was admirably prepared for the work, was appointed. No one except Dr. Jex-Blake wanted the post. Certainly Mrs. Garrett Anderson did not, and Mrs. Thorne, in accepting it, had to give up her medical career. She had been a matriculated student in medicine for years and, while this training was to be of much use for her future work, to relinquish her profession was a sacrifice. Undoubtedly, Dr. Jex-Blake had expected the post. She had looked forward to the day when, as a

The London School of Medicine for Women

qualified medical woman, the control of the school would pass into her hands. The entries in her diary are brief and generous. 'About the best possible,' she wrote in regard to Mrs. Thorne's appointment. 'With her excellent sense and perfect temper. So much better than I.'[1] None the less, the hurt was deep. She changed her plans and forthwith decided to go to Edinburgh to practise. For some years her connection with the London School of Medicine for Women lasted, but she seldom attended committees. When in 1883 Mr. Norton resigned the post of dean, she made a rare appearance at the council to vote, as a minority of one, against the appointment of Mrs. Garrett Anderson. In 1896 when the school was to be rebuilt and the council proposed to borrow part of the Oakes bequest for building purposes, she objected and ceased to be a trustee.

S.J.-B. to Mrs. I. Thorne   Edinburgh, 6 May 1897
'I feel that I have no alternative but to resign my position as one of the trustees of the London School. I disapprove of the action taken as to expenditure without the money in hand and also to the incorporation of the school at this crisis; and as no attention has been paid to my suggestion that the question should be submitted to the whole Governing Body I can but free myself from all responsibility in the matter. You will please report my resignation to the Executive Council.'

[1] Dr. Margaret Todd's *Life of Sophia Jex-Blake.*

The London School of Medicine for Women

At the next meeting of the governing body, Mrs. Garrett Anderson proposed the resolution: 'The governors of the London School of Medicine for Women desire in accepting Dr. Sophia Jex-Blake's resignation to record their appreciation of the great value of her services in the foundation and early organization of the School and their sincere regret that she differs from the executive council in the view of the measures which in their judgment have become necessary in consequence of the fact that the School has again outgrown the accommodation of the present premises.' The Dean added that in the early years she had been timid and considered the time had not arrived for establishing a separate school of medicine for women. To organize a school on the slender sum raised by Dr. Jex-Blake required great optimism and she thought the idea of rebuilding the school was a far less hazardous proceeding, but she and Dr. Jex-Blake had changed places, for she was hopeful that the money could now be raised while Dr. Jex-Blake was fearful of the financial risk involved.

Mrs. Garrett Anderson was forty-seven when in 1883 she succeeded Mr. Norton as dean. She held the post for twenty years and then became president until her death in 1917; indeed, for more than thirty years the school cannot have been far from her thoughts. When she took office its initial difficulties had been solved, and from

1883 onwards the school, guided, led and inspired by her, made steady progress. It was enlarged, rebuilt and transformed from a small two-storied house into a college of the University of London. By precept and example she taught the students the ethics of the medical profession. 'The first thing women must learn', she had said years ago, 'is to behave like gentlemen.' She left the impress of her character on hundreds of students who worked under her. Her particular gifts were just those which the school at that stage needed from its leader. She was vigorous in mind and body, overflowing with energy: she did not shrink from responsibility; she inspired confidence in a wide circle; her judgment was good; she was fair; she had a business head and shone at a committee, bringing forward well-considered ideas but not laying down the law. She had dignity; she could be stern but usually she was accessible, urbane and charitable in judgment; the people with whom she worked became friends. Her courage was infectious. Perhaps her principal defect as dean was that she could not remember the students. Their names and faces passed her by and as their numbers increased, so did her difficulty. However, her goodwill embraced them all and possibly they did not guess how hard she found it to put the right name even to the last gold medallist.

In 1883 the school building was in essentials as it had been nine years before when it passed into the hands of the council. An iron shed had been added in the garden

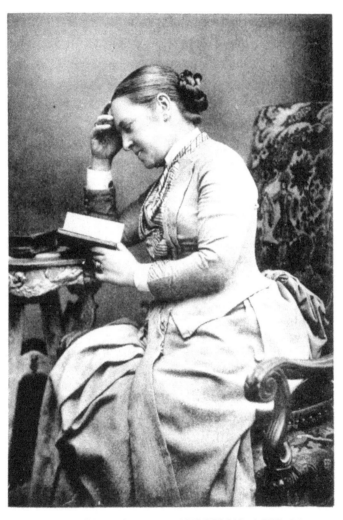

ELIZABETH GARRETT ANDERSON, AGED 54

as a lecture-room. It was unsightly and uncomfortable—
an oven in summer and a noisy ice-house in winter with
rain on the corrugated iron roof. Anatomy arrangements were primitive. Research was impossible, for
laboratories did not exist. There were few facilities and
no amenities, but in spite of all this hardship, or perhaps
as a result of it, the students did conspicuously well.
There were thirty-seven medical women on the register
and forty students in the school and hospital.

For years poverty oppressed the council. Fees from
students did not nearly cover the working expenses of
the school. One of the reports about this time noted,
'all that was needed to make the school a complete success was a larger entry of students.' True—but the building did not attract them and could not hold them. It was
too expensive to give all courses of lectures simultane-
ously, but spread over three years the curriculum could
be completed. How could the council improve the
school? The Dean was a 'good beggar' and the sums of
money which year by year she collected for the school,
at first to cover the deficit in current budgets and later
to supplement the various building funds, would have
been remarkable if the school had been her only care,
but this was not so.

The New Hospital for Women was growing fast and
made insistent claims for larger and better accommodation during the same period, 1890 to 1900. Friends of
the women's movement represented a select but small

part of the public; few of them were rich, although for years they helped the school and hospital continuously and generously, while Mrs. Anderson led the appeals and collected most of the money. In the subscription lists the same names appear constantly.

The year after Mrs. Garrett Anderson became dean was the tenth anniversary of the foundation of the school. A celebration had to mark the occasion. The council decided to hold a conversazione and the sum of £10 was voted from the school funds while the students contributed £11 10s. for an awning, and a 'very success-ful' party took place. 'If I give a party,' said the Dean to one of the students, 'it is a good one.' Certainly she loved entertaining and excelled at it. Whether the party was a private one or an official gathering, none of the guests enjoyed themselves more than their hostess, who radiated pleasure upon the company.

In spite of discomforts and lack of apparatus, the level of instruction at the school must have been high. As soon as examining boards consented to receive them, the women students won for their school gold medals, ex-hibitions and honours. At the Irish University Miss Fleury carried everything before her; on one occasion, like Miss Agnata Ramsay in the Classical Tripos at Cambridge 1887, she surpassed other candidates to such an extent that she occupied a class by herself. One of the early duties of the new dean was to present for gradua-tion Mrs. Scharlieb and Miss Shove, the first women

The London School of Medicine for Women

medical students to qualify at the University of London. This happy occasion was a contrast to the discomfort Elizabeth and her father had experienced in 1862, when after great labour their petition to the University had been rejected. Then by a majority of one, the University had refused to accept women for examination. Mr. Newson Garrett was growing old, but no one rejoiced more than he over the new world into which women had entered.

His daughter wrote to him:

E.G.A. to N.G. *London, 6 May 1883*
'The first ladies who have earned the medical degree of the London University will be presented for graduation next Wednesday 2 p.m. at Burlington House. I am to have the honour of presenting them to Lord Granville as I am now Dean of the Medical School for Women. I think in memory of our efforts 21 years ago you should come up for it.'

Mr. Garrett attended the ceremony.

In his address, the Chancellor alluded to Mrs. Scharlieb's record—a gold medal, a scholarship and two examinations passed in the first division. The high attainment of the early students continued. In the same year Mr. Norton said of the class examinations in surgery, 'They are the best papers I have ever received at any examination.' In 1889 in the opening address at the University of Glasgow, Professor George Buchanan

233

said, 'more than half of the honours of the University of London in anatomy, physiology and materia medica were taken by women as against all comers, from all schools.'

Naturally, in the early days, medicine attracted eccentric as well as able women. A pink flannel coat, scalloped round the edge like a dressing-jacket, appeared in the lecture-room, and for dissecting, evening dresses were used after they had passed their prime and could not grace a conversazione again. Some of the most brilliant students were preparing to be missionaries and their devotion and outlook transformed work into a crusade. From the first, the Dean set her face against supplying 'a little medical knowledge to missionaries'. They had to take the course or to stay away. More than once she said that she 'distrusted the capacity of most people to be efficient in two professions'. She looked upon medicine as a profession and not a charity. She thought the willingness of women to sacrifice themselves had been exploited. Some worldly wisdom would be good for a change and she preferred the students, when qualified, to practise in England and to earn good incomes. The mission field meant exile, penury and a bad climate: possibly illness and early death. Yet some medical missionaries were the women she most admired.

The advent of medical women to India, which began while Mr. Norton was dean, is mentioned in the *Indian Female Evangelist*, 29 October 1881. The Maharajah of a native state applied to Miss Beilby, a medical missionary in Lucknow, for medical attendance on his wife—who being in *purdah* could not see a male doctor. A cure was effected after many weeks' residence in the state, where Dr. Beilby was the only European. Before leaving she was desired to appear before the Maharanee. She was received in her private room. The attendants were dismissed. The Maharanee charged Dr. Beilby to take a message to the Great Queen to tell her of the cruel sufferings of Indian women. 'Write it small, Doctor Miss,' said she, 'for I want to put it in a locket'.

The Queen received Dr. Beilby and desired it to be made known that she sympathized with every effort to relieve the sufferings of Indian women. Did Her Majesty realize what this entailed? Relief to native women could come only from qualified medical practitioners of their own sex, and the one training school for them in the Empire was the London School of Medicine for Women. No one is consistent, not even the greatest of queens. For the women of India the help of medical women was essential, but the idea of women practising medicine in Great Britain distressed Queen Victoria. Indeed, some weeks after the incident of the locket, the Queen's private physician announced that the royal patronage would be withdrawn from an international medical congress held in London if medical women were admitted, and so the women were shut out.

In the following year Queen Victoria made a friendly

gesture to medical women. Mrs. Scharlieb was received by Her Majesty at Windsor and by the Prince and Princess of Wales at Marlborough House before she left to take up professional work in Madras. The following year, Dr. Edith Pechey and Dr. Hitchcock started work in Bombay, where, by the generosity of a Parsee, Mr. Cama, a splendid hospital had been built for the treatment of native women by women. The Government accepted responsibility for its upkeep and Dr. Pechey was gazetted as physician-in-charge. Her influence proved important and a pamphlet which she wrote later on child marriage was translated into many dialects and widely circulated. Some years later she had the unprecedented honour of being appointed a member of the Senate of the University of Bombay.

In 1885, through the Countess of Dufferin, practical measures were taken in India when, as wife to the Viceroy, she started the association for the supply of Female Medical Service to the Women of India.

Year by year the London School of Medicine progressed and the number of students increased. The alliance between the Royal Free Hospital and the School was completely successful. Every fifth year the agreement was renewed and mutual compliments paid. Once a year Mrs. Anderson entertained the students. In 1881 before she became dean, she wrote to Mrs. Newson Garrett: 'We have a students' supper which will mount up to a pretty large party, probably 70 or 80, all to a sit down supper.' In 1889, as dean, she gave an evening party to two hundred where, 'Corney Grain was even better than usual. Part of the affair was a take-off of two fashionable doctors, Andrew Clark and another. Sir Andrew Clark, who was one of the guests, enjoyed the fun as much as any one present.'

In 1891 Miss Julia Cock, M.D., became sub-dean. It was a happy arrangement for the school and for the officers. A partnership of outstanding harmony followed between the dean and sub-dean. Miss Cock had the vision of a statesman and her loyalty to the dean was that of real friendship. She insisted that all the limelight should fall on Mrs. Garrett Anderson, while she did the drudgery. Her organization for the students was particularly valuable. She gave them self-government as far as possible, a plan which worked admirably. Under their joint leadership the school was transformed. In 1885 and again in 1891 and 1892 the leases of adjacent small houses were bought, at a cost of from one thousand to two thousand pounds each. They were in bad repair and the ground landlords objected to practical anatomy on their property. Mrs. Thorne, the honorary secretary, dealt effectively with these difficulties.

In 1893 Miss L. B. Aldrich Blake, after a brilliant career as a student, was appointed curator of the museum at the Royal Free Hospital—the first appointment there to be held by a qualified medical woman.

In 1896 the unprecedented entry of fifty new students

compelled the dean and council to face the question of rebuilding. An iron shed and extra little houses would not meet the case. A new site for the school was first considered, and when none suitable could be found, the council decided to rebuild on the existing site, at an estimated cost of £20,000. One block of buildings would follow another, and meantime, as best they might, teachers and students would continue their work. By this time students' fees covered the working expenses and for the building fund the council proposed to borrow £3,700 from the school's endowments and for the balance to arrange a bank loan. As a result of a letter from the Dean to *The Times* of 11 December 1897, over £1,600 was collected.

A building lease for eighty years was granted by the ground landlords and the work proceeded. When the first new block was ready the school was honoured by visits from T.R.H. the Prince and Princess of Wales (11 July 1898).

The Prince came first by himself and went over the New Hospital and the School with the Dean, charming every one.

Two years later Mrs. Anderson wrote to her father:

E.G.A. to N.G.   4 Upper Berkeley St., 16 Oct. 1900
'We have had another splendid donation this week. £5,000 for the School! It came to me, or rather the letter promising it, yesterday morning. The only con-

dition imposed is that we are not to borrow any more
money till the entire debt is paid off. We shall hope now
gradually to make up the rest. The kind donor is not, I
think, a very rich man. His father, Mr. Turle, was for
many years organist at Westminster Abbey. He was at
the opening of the School a fortnight ago, and I spoke
then of the heavy debt on the building and how thankful
we should be to get rid of some of it. The words apparently went home.'

In 1901 the school became one of the colleges of the
newly constituted University of London. The following
year its qualified students began to hold posts at the
Royal Free Hospital such as surgical and medical regis-
trars, anaesthetists and resident medical officers. Appointments to the honorary visiting staff soon followed.

In 1903 Mrs. Garrett Anderson, at the age of sixty-
seven, resigned the office of dean and Miss Cock succeeded her with Miss Aldrich Blake as sub-dean—
another happy and effective combination. Mrs. Garrett
Anderson became president, an office created in her
honour.

She and her husband moved to Aldeburgh and from
there, despite the trials of a journey by the Great Eastern
Railway, she often came to the school, attending committees and rarely missing social functions.

In 1908 technical education was made eligible for a
parliamentary grant and no time was lost by the dean,

The London School of Medicine for Women

Miss Cock, and the secretary, Miss L. M. Brooks, in proving to Sir George Newman, then at the Board of Education, that medical training was technical.

The women's school was the first medical school to apply for a grant and received the first payment of £169 in 1911. In the years that followed the increasing grants from the Treasury became an important part of the school income and financial anxiety ceased.

In 1913 the President supported a further building scheme and promised £1,000 a year for three years. Drawing the cheques pleased her greatly. H.M. Queen Mary opened this extension in 1916. In 1914 Miss Cock died and Miss Aldrich Blake became dean. By this time the school was in its stride. As president, Mrs. Garrett Anderson lavished thought and love on it. Among her last words were: 'We must not desert the School.' It was developed and rebuilt by her and guided from youth to maturity.

10

THE NEW HOSPITAL FOR WOMEN

>>➤➾●⊂≺≺

In 1866 Miss Garrett, L.S.A., at last licensed to practise, was able to plan her professional career. In addition to her private work she started the St. Mary's Dispensary for Women, Seymour Place, to enable women to obtain medical and surgical treatment from qualified medical practitioners of their own sex. The crowded district of Lisson Grove was close at hand. St. Mary's Hospital, about a mile away, was the nearest general hospital. The Rev. J. Llewelyn Davies as rector of the parish welcomed the dispensary; the site was well chosen. For several years Miss Garrett was the only visiting physician and at first she also acted as dispenser. She attended out-patients three times a week, visited patients in their own homes and took charge of midwifery cases in the neighbourhood.

From the first, the dispensary had an eminent consulting staff. Dr. Hughlings Jackson and Dr. Broadbent were consulting physicians, and Mr. Critchett, Mr. Thomas Smith and Mr. A. T. Norton acted on the surgical side. Its popularity was unquestioned. Patients[1] crowded the little rooms. That they were asked to pay small fees did not deter them. They paid willingly in order to be treated by a woman. By 1871 9,000 names were on the dispensary books and more than 40,000 visits had been paid, whilst 250 midwifery cases had been attended in their own homes. A colleague, Miss Morgan, M.D. Zürich (afterwards Mrs. Hoggan), now helped Mrs. Anderson. Unfortunately her degree was a foreign one and she could not put her name on the Medical Register. It was irregular but inevitable.

Some patients were seriously ill and some had journeyed from the country. The need for beds was great. A committee was formed, and friends such as the Rev. Llewelyn Davies and Mr. Plaskitt were original and important members.

In 1872 ten beds were provided over the old out-patient department and the dispensary was renamed the New Hospital for Women. The Earl of Shaftesbury, K.G., opened the ward. A higher fee of sixpence per visit was charged, but, undeterred, patients thronged the rooms. The New Hospital for Women was more than a philanthropic effort. It helped to solve one of the social questions of the day by showing what trained women could do, principally by giving them experience in responsible medical and surgical work, and also by

[1] Within the first few weeks 60 to 90 women and children attended on each consulting afternoon.

employing them as clerk, secretary and dispenser.

It won professional success as well as popularity. It proved that women for certain ailments preferred to consult medical women and that women doctors were efficient. By 1874 the pressure of work demanded larger premises. The leases of two and then three houses, numbers 220, 222 and 224 in the Marylebone Road, were bought. At first the third house was sub-let but the others, with their boards well scrubbed and plenty of iodoform everywhere, provided accommodation for twenty-six beds. In the following year the transfer was made. The new building seemed palatial after the house in Seymour Place. It consisted of unpretentious houses facing south with strips of garden leading to the Marylebone Road, and it stood where the Great Central Railway Hotel was built later. A small and very generous public upheld Mrs. Garrett Anderson, but £3,555 10s. had been spent and a debt of £500 weighed on the minds of the committee. However by 1876 this debt and the dilapidations on the Seymour Place house had been paid, while a third physician, Mrs. Louisa Atkins, M.D. Zürich, had joined the staff and a resident pupil was installed.

For nearly twenty years Mrs. Garrett Anderson was the only member of the staff who would undertake serious surgical work. She knew the limits of her training. Each operation caused her intense anxiety, but she insisted that medical women should do the professional work of the hospital. Disagreement over this point arose with one of her colleagues. Indeed, Mrs. Hoggan fell from grace by urging that Dr. Meredith, an operating gynaecologist of experience, should be invited to undertake all the abdominal surgery. 'No men or no hospital' represented Mrs. Anderson's view, and with the help of the surgeons on her consulting staff carried the point which she considered vital—that all the professional work of the hospital should be done by qualified medical women. Mrs. Hoggan resigned in 1876. In the hospital report for 1878 it was recorded that the operation of ovariotomy had been performed twice by a member of the staff (Mrs. Anderson). 'The committee are not aware of this formidable operation having been ever before, in Europe at least, successfully performed by a woman.' It was regarded as a most serious operation and one not to be attempted in the hospital since the death of the patient would injure its reputation. For the first case Mrs. Anderson rented part of a private house. The rooms were cleaned and redecorated with fresh paint and whitewash, and the patient and her nurses installed. Sir Thomas Smith (of St. Bartholomew's Hospital) helped at the operation, which was successful. All went well, but Mr. Anderson, who met the cost of the rooms and of their preparation, remarked: 'We shall be in the bankruptcy court if Elizabeth's surgical practice increases.' The second case remained in the hospital and gradually confidence was established, but Mrs. Anderson never enjoyed operating and she was delighted when skilled women surgeons relieved her of this side of the hospital practice.

As the years passed other medical women joined the staff of the New Hospital and with the passage of the Russell Gurney Enabling Act and the opening of qualifying examinations to women, irregularities in regard to the degrees held by the staff ceased. By 1885 there were four visiting physicians attached to the hospital, Mrs. Marshall, Mrs. de la Cherois and Mrs. Atkins, in addition to Mrs. Garrett Anderson. In the spring of that year Mrs. Anderson went to Australia with her husband and children, and during her absence left Mrs. Mary Scharlieb in charge of the surgical beds. After a distinguished career as a student at the London School of Medicine for Women, Mrs. Scharlieb had practised in India, gaining a great reputation for surgical and obstetrical skill. At that time no other woman had had a similar training in abdominal surgery and probably few surgeons equalled her skill, her slender hands seeming to go everywhere with marvellous speed.

Many references occur in Mrs. Anderson's letters to the operations she was obliged to do during the first twenty years of hospital practice. In 1886, writing to her husband who was in America, she said: 'my patient is doing excellently. It turned out to be a very uncommon case and I have offered the tumour to the Museum of the College of Surgeons as [Sir Spencer] Wells says they have only one like it.' Again in 1889 in a letter to Mrs. Garrett: 'I have had an operation which I had never done before or seen done and which is more often than not fatal.' And on 25 July 1889: 'Both the cases at 222 have done quite well, which as I was entirely without outside help is a great comfort. I shall leave them to-morrow practically convalescent.'

In 1887 the leases of the premises in Marylebone Road had expired and as a renewal could not be arranged another site had to be found or other private houses bought and transformed into a hospital. An extensive search in the neighbourhood of the Euston Road followed and, finally, in 1888, the seventy-year lease of a site opposite St. Pancras Church was bought for £3,000. The freehold was available and the committee intended to buy it when funds permitted. Meanwhile the contract for the new building amounted to £13,584. For twenty-two years, without appeal to the public, hospital work on an increasing scale had been done. Now it was felt that a public appeal must be made to provide a building fund. This was launched at a meeting at the Mansion House to which Miss Florence Nightingale sent a contribution of fifty pounds. 'You want efficient women doctors,' she wrote, 'for India most of all whose native women are now our sisters, our charge. There are at least 40 million who will only have women doctors and who have none.' The Committee aimed at collecting £20,000 to defray the cost of the site and building.

The New Hospital for Women

On 7 May 1888 H.R.H. the Princess of Wales (later Queen Alexandra), accompanied by the Prince of Wales and the young Princesses Victoria and Maud, laid the foundation stone at 144 Euston Road. By 1889 £11,241 had been collected, leaving a balance of £9,000 still to be found. A series of drawing-room meetings was arranged by Mrs. Anderson, Mrs. Scharlieb and Mrs. Marshall, at which collecting cards for £5, £10 and £20 were distributed. Mrs. Anderson spoke at thirty-seven of these meetings. On 2 March 1889 she wrote to Mrs. Garrett, 'our drawing-room meetings are going off successfully. In the two this week, both small ones, we have got rid of twenty-one £20 cards and several smaller ones and they have all been thoroughly interested in my "story". About eight more meetings are already organized and some will be very large,' and again on 23 March 1889 to Mrs. Garrett she reported: 'We have had a busy week with meetings. We have placed more than £1,000 worth of cards. We had one donation of £300 paid into our account without a word by a Mr. Vallance whom none of us know.' On 6 July she wrote to Mrs. Garrett: 'We are now into our eighteenth £1,000 so if 50 people bring in £20 each we are all right.' On 12 July 1889 seven hundred invitations were sent to card-holders for a party in Mrs. Anderson's house. They had collected £21,200, including a donation of £1,000 from Mr. Tate. 'It is a splendid result and every one was much pleased.' Without a pause Mrs. Anderson began to organize a bazaar for the autumn. She meant this to complete the sum required for the new building and it did so.

In 1888 Mrs. Anderson, Mrs. Marshall, and Mrs. de la Cherois were on the in-patient and Miss Cock, Mrs. Scharlieb, and Miss Walker on the out-patient staff of the hospital. The new building provided forty-two beds and an ophthalmic department under the direction of Miss Charlotte Ellaby, M.D. It was estimated that the cost of maintenance would rise from £2,000 as in the past at 222 Marylebone Road to £3,000 annually. Four years later, 1892, when the hospital was steering a straight course for long and useful service, Mrs. Garrett Anderson resigned her position on the visiting staff. The managing committee stated that to her 'indomitable energy and ability the hospital owes—not only its foundation and its great and continuous success, but to her is owing the recognition and established position of medical women in England'. Resolutions such as this are not taken on oath, but probably this one expressed conviction.

Mrs. Scharlieb and Miss Julia Cock were promoted to in-patient service, and under the former the surgical reputation of the hospital forged ahead, while Miss Cock proved an admirable clinical teacher.

In 1896 Mrs. Russell Gurney died and left a substantial legacy to the hospital. Mrs. Anderson referred to this gift in the hospital report and her mind went back to the beginning of the movement for training women in medicine. 'It would have been difficult in the early days to have found in London two more honoured names than theirs [Mr. and Mrs. Russell Gurney] or two from whose countenance a new and untried movement could gain more substantial support in the judgment of thoughtful people.'

After leaving the active staff Mrs. Anderson's interest in the hospital continued and she reported to Mrs. Garrett the pleasant words of Sir Thomas Smith about its work.

E.G.A. to Mrs. N.G.   *17 March 1900*

'We have had a most successful annual meeting for the New. Sir Thomas Smith, the eminent surgeon, has been coming a good deal (some 25 or 30 times) to see big operations at the New and he spoke and said how extremely good he thought the surgical work was and that indeed it could not be better. After the speaking was over a gentleman in the audience promised £400 for the debt on the new operating-room so Sir T.S.'s praise bore immediate and excellent fruit. The good donor is a Mr. Turle, son of the late organist at Westminster Abbey.'

When Mrs. Anderson resigned the office of chairman to the hospital committee, she introduced as her successor Mr. A. G. Pollock, who served for twenty-five years, presiding over one improvement after another until age told on him. He felt himself unable to continue the work or to hand it to any one except the son of the woman at whose wish he began his long and generous service. And so for a spell Alan Anderson came to the hospital as chairman, until it started fairly on its new course, first under Sophy, Lady Hall, and now under Lady Robertson.

At Mrs. Anderson's death in 1917 the name of the hospital was altered and it became the 'Elizabeth Garrett Anderson Hospital'; since then devoted workers have served it well, enlarging and improving it out of recognition. It remains invaluable as a training ground for medical women in responsible medicine and surgery, and the patients, whether in the hospital itself or at the Rosa Morison Home of Recovery at Barnet, purchased for the hospital in 1913 by a legacy from Miss Morison, testify to their appreciation of its service. It now has 105 beds and its latest appeal was launched on the centenary of Elizabeth Garrett's birth, 9 June 1936, to provide adequate quarters for the nursing staff. The hospital is a living memorial to its founder and those who worked with her.

11

THE BRITISH MEDICAL
ASSOCIATION

ᐳᐳᐳᐸᐸᐸ

When Elizabeth Garrett qualified in 1865, she considered herself eligible for membership of the British
Medical Association but other matters occupied her and
she did not apply for admission until eight years later.

She looked forward to the time when other qualified
women would be in the profession. Membership of the
British Medical Association would be of value to them.
To be excluded would be a stigma. At branch meetings
doctors met on friendly terms; professional difficulties
and experiences might be discussed; the papers on medical subjects were useful. In a sense, the Association was
a trade union. It protected the rights and safeguarded
the interests of medical practitioners, and it guided members in the observance of correct professional conduct.
The ethics of the profession and its courtesies had to be
learnt by young doctors and their best school was the
Association.

In 1873 Mrs. Anderson's nomination paper, influen-
tially signed, was accepted by the Paddington Branch of

the British Medical Association. Two years passed before the fact of her membership became widely known. Criticism of the admission of a woman to the British Medical Association was voiced at the annual general meeting in Edinburgh 1875. Mrs. Garrett Anderson had attended the meeting in order to read a paper in the obstetrical section. The storm which burst on her was unexpected. It was said that a 'liberty' had been taken. Professor Christison was president. His antagonism to medical women had reached white heat over the claims of Miss Jex-Blake and her friends and at the date of this meeting their struggle in Edinburgh was recent history. Mr. Pemberton (Birmingham) led the attack. Mrs. Anderson's 'best counsellor' was not at hand but she wrote to him frequently.

E.G.A. to J.G.S.A.   *Edinburgh, 4 Aug. 1875*
'Storms are brewing here. Yesterday we applied for tickets, mine as a member was given at once but Mary's [Mrs. Marshall, M.D.] claim for a student's ticket was met by the assertion that all these had been given away long ago. However we saw the chief secretary and I said it would be so much more comfortable to me if Mary could be with me upon which he good-naturedly gave her a ticket. However before the first general meeting some hours later he sent Mary a note to say he found he had exceeded his powers and begging her not to use the ticket till further notice, he would do all he could

to get the matter arranged. So I went alone to the President's address [Christison's]. It was horribly dull and long and was medico-political rather than medical. I was the only woman present as the Hoggans have not yet come. When it ended some general business was gone thro' (I had left to be in time for M. Duncan's dinner 7) and into this a man named Pemberton introduced the subject of women members by moving that a vote of the general body of the Association be taken as to the admission of women. It was ruled by 35 to 33 that his motion was out of order and could not be brought forward then. He gave notice that he would bring it forward again at a general meeting (there is one of these each day) and he will probably do so to-day or to-morrow. If he carries his motion and an appeal is made to the Association it is quite certain what their answer will be. E. Hart [Dr. Ernest Hart, Editor, *British Medical Journal*] says I ought to be on the watch for Pemberton's motion and be ready to speak against it. I wish your wise counsels, beloved, were within reach. I should like to know what you would advise. I don't want to fail as a leader even of a forlorn hope but it grates against my taste making anything of a self-defensive speech to such a body. If I do speak I will try to lift the question on to a higher plane and to appeal to the best part of their minds. I must get on to Arthur's Seat and try to see my way to doing this. They can scarcely shut the door against other women without also turning

me out, which is so far a good thing as many would pull
up at this. I shall perhaps write you again later, dearest,
if there is anything to say. Dr. Struthers and Wm. Marshall are here and are very kind and nice. They breakfast
with us to-morrow. My paper will not be read to-day
certainly, and I should think very likely not at all. Don't
think I am unhappy, dearest. I am serious—as in the
sight of a battle one must be—and I think there are a
thousand chances to one that I shall be utterly and completely defeated but this is all in the day's work. Some
one must do it and with all my inner joys (you and the
dear babies and my work) I can stand it better than most
people could. If I can do my duty the defeat will be but
one more step towards final victory.'

A few hours later she wrote again:

E.G.A. to J.G.S.A.   *Edinburgh, 4 Aug. 1875*
'After posting my letter this morning we were caught
by callers and in consequence did not get to the meeting
before the general meeting of the day had begun. The
room and even the passage leading to it were so cramful
that we gave up all attempt at getting in. We had been
told that Pemberton's motion would not likely be
brought on to-day. However it was and tho' we have
not heard any particulars the tone of the meeting was
evidently strongly against us. The secretary had this
morning given Mary leave to use her ticket, but after
this debate he sent a messenger here post haste to beg

that she would not. However as we did not come home
to lunch this was never received and we both spent the
afternoon in the sections hearing various papers and discussions. So I have missed the opportunity of saying
anything. To-night there is a reception and there we
shall hear more particulars. I fancy it is all but certain
they will not allow our [Mrs. Hoggan's and E.G.A.'s]
papers to be read or even taken as read. I can't tell you
whether it will be worth while waiting till Saturday. I
shall only do so if it seems likely to be of some use. It
strikes me as very unfair to have brought up the discussion to-day without formal notice. But for gossip I
should not have heard of the threatened attack at all. I
send a little word to Louie.'

After two days of suspense Mrs. Anderson was
allowed to read her paper.

E.G.A. to J.G.S.A.   *Edinburgh, 6 Aug. 1875*
'We have had a great triumph! The paper was very
well received, heard by an immense audience and a vote
of thanks passed by acclamation. I do hope it will be
useful in a solid way to the cause. On Wednesday all
looked black and I heard that positively the paper would
not be read. Yesterday too it was not down. After much
consultation with Mary and mainly by her advice I went
to see some of the heads of my section, Keiller and M.
Duncan, and told them that I thought I was being badly
used in the paper being suppressed on any ground but

demerit. I said to them if they would say to me that any one of their number had read it and thought it not worth producing I would at once acquiesce in the decision but that I did not think it ought to be stopped in deference to prejudice. My visits had some effect for in the afternoon I had a message to say it would be put down for to-day. The room was crammed and every one shook hands afterwards till I was reminded of St. Pancras and School Board meetings. Love to all, dearest, I am called away.'

In spite of the opposition of the meeting towards the admission of women Mrs. Garrett Anderson's election to the British Medical Association was legal and could not be annulled. Mrs. Hoggan, however, who had been elected the previous year, was discovered to be unregistered, possessing only the degree M.D. Zürich, and her election was stated to be irregular. A hundred men in the same plight were re-elected but Mrs. Hoggan was not. The following resolution was carried: 'That it be an instruction to the Secretary, between now and the next Annual Meeting, to issue a circular addressed to every member of the association requesting an opinion, Yes or No, as to the admission of female practitioners to membership.'

The result of this plebiscite of the Home Association, then numbering 6,230, was not obtained for some time. Out of 4,161 replies, 3,072 were against and 1,051 in favour of admitting qualified medical women to membership. This vote had no legal force but it encouraged the council to bring forward a resolution definitely excluding women at the annual meeting in 1878, held at Bath. The President proposed to add a clause to the Articles of Association: 'That no female shall be eligible as a member of the Association.' Dr. Wade moved and Dr. A. P. Stewart, 'as the original culprit', since he had proposed Mrs. Garrett Anderson's nomination in 1873, seconded the resolution. After speeches on both sides, Mrs. Garrett Anderson rose and 'was received with loud cheers'. An abstract from the excellent report in the *British Medical Journal*, August 1878, follows. She said:

'Mr. President and Gentlemen, I shall treat this question from an entirely impersonal point of view and I shall not say a word as to the disadvantage to women practitioners if they are not allowed to become members of the Association. I look upon it that you are entirely against my side but that, in this view, you are entirely impersonal (cheers), that it is with you a question of public medical policy whether women in the profession should be allowed to enter into any share of this great Association and it seems to me that our side should be fully put before you.' She continued: 'The first question is, what are the objects of the Association? Are those right who describe it as a social club? In its Articles of Association its objects are said to be the promotion of medical science, and the promotion of the interests of the profession and of fellowship. Will either of these be forwarded by excluding medical women? Science cannot gain by refusing evidence from witnesses who upon some points are specially qualified to give it. Moreover if the Association exists to promote medical science it ought to aim at promoting it generally and not partially. If women are *bona fide* members of the profession they have a right to claim that the Association should not be indifferent about their advance as well as that of the rest of the body, it should be wished that every fresh wave of progress in medical knowledge should carry them as well as the men forward. So with regard to the second object of the Association, the promotion of the interests of the profession—women as well as men now being in the medical profession their interests should be cared for, and every care should be taken to make them share in the corporate interest of the body. No one wishes medical women to set at nought the common or unwritten laws of the profession, to be willing to do any amount of work for the lowest prices, or to disregard the courtesies of medical etiquette, and how can they be expected to develop a spirit of comradeship, of regard for the common weal, if they are not permitted to enjoy even the most limited amount of professional fellowship? Then again, there is the social element in the Association. Though not in its essence a club it is true that one valuable purpose of the Association is that of bringing those together whose corporate interests are identical but whose individual interests often clash. It would be Utopian to say that mutual knowledge would always make people friendly but it is true that enthusiastic dislikes are maintained with greater difficulty between those who are personally acquainted with each other. Medical men do not dislike each other half so much as they dislike medical women and there is, therefore, the more need that they should be brought, as regards medical men, under the mollifying influences of social intercourse. We all know the story of Charles Lamb. He had been heaping abuse on the head of some one, when his friend said: "Lamb, how can you say that? How can you hate so heartily a man you do not know?" The answer was: "My dear fellow, of course I do not know him. How could I hate him at all if I did?" (Cheers). All these arguments however are based upon the theory that from henceforth medical women will form an appreciable part of the profession, and considering that the Legislature has spoken in favour of their claims, that the highest examining body in the Kingdom has consented to examine them, that a complete school of medicine with the clinical practice of a large general hospital, a museum and a library, have been organized for the exclusive use of female students and that the School has £12,000 in its exchequer, it is not likely that the movement, having survived its initial difficulties, will now die—eight English women are now on the Medical Register and every year will see the numbers considerably increased. The reasons assigned for keeping women out of the Association are first, that there is a moral impropriety in discussing medical questions in the presence of men and women and second, that certain eminent members of the Association threaten to resign if women are allowed to remain.' The first of these two arguments Mrs. Anderson wished to approach with great respect. It seemed to her that there was absolutely nothing opposed to true refinement in men and women who are working constantly at the same subjects meeting from time to time and talking over their work. Considering how much of the practice of every doctor concerns women, it is incredible that they find it impossible to speak upon medical topics in the presence of medical women. To Mrs. Anderson it seemed that 'the study of medicine and surgery does not even *approach the confines* of indelicacy'. 'No doubt there are in surgery,' she continued, 'two or three subjects in the discussion of which it would offend good taste for women to be present, but as medical women in England practise exclusively among women and children and the subjects in question relate only to men, it is in the last degree improbable that women would even wish to be present, and the remote contingency is one which could easily be guarded against. It is much to be regretted no doubt if any eminent members secede from the association, but it is possible to buy even gold too dearly. A great Association like the British Medical does not grow and flourish by the support of even the most valued names, but by keeping true to its largest purposes, and these are in our case the promotion of science and the promotion of fellowship. The issue before you is this. Shall the Association continue to act in harmony with those purposes? Shall it continue to keep itself in accord with the facts by recognizing as it has recognized for five years the existence of medical women? or shall it break off from all its own best traditions by refusing fellowship to members of the profession not in themselves unworthy of it? Shall it decide to commit in a moment of reactionary excitement an act of hostility in itself useless, and sure to be hereafter regretted, against a movement the strength and vitality of which cannot be doubted?' (Cheers.)

Dr. J. Ford Anderson, who was present, recorded his impressions. 'The effect of Mrs. Anderson's personality and her impersonal and pleasant speech produced a transformation scene in the meeting she had addressed. One member after another rose and protested that they were charmed and any action they might take would be entirely on the principles involved.' The meeting then voted on the motion: 'No female shall be eligible for election as a member of the Association.' The vote was not to be retrospective. By show of hands there was a majority for the motion.

Following this event, for nineteen years Mrs. Garrett Anderson remained the only woman member of the British Medical Association. She attended branch and annual meetings and usually spoke. She joined in discussions and generally went to the social functions in connection with annual meetings. Hostility pervaded the atmosphere. 'Sometimes the feeling of disapproval becomes almost unbearable,' she wrote. All her courage was needed. Her sister-in-law, Mrs. Marshall, M.D., went with her as a guest and her presence helped, but still, to a sensitive person the ordeal was great.

Gradually the ice thawed and in 1892 at the annual general meeting of the Association in Nottingham, the hostile clause was expunged by an overwhelming majority. In a meeting of three hundred members, three or four only voted for its continuance. To Dr. J. H. Galton and other friends this result may be attributed, but there is no doubt that Mrs. Anderson's character had had its effect. The vote was confirmed shortly afterwards at a second general meeting in London. By this time the number of medical women on the Register had risen to 135, as compared with eight in 1875.

In 1896 the East Anglian Branch of the British Medical Association elected Mrs. Garrett Anderson as their president for the year 1896-7, an honour she appreciated. Her friend, Dr. Michael Beverley of Norwich, enthusiastically supported her election and helped her in the duties involved. He and she were keen gardeners and, when they did not discuss professional matters, the herbaceous border and the water garden afforded them ample scope. Mrs. Garrett Anderson's address as presi-

dent began with these words: 'My first duty is to thank
you most heartily for the honour I am receiving at your
hands. To be invited to preside over the senior branch
of your Association would in any case be a great and
valued distinction and the honour in my case is enhanced
by the fact that it has been given by my own country-
men, by those among whom my family has lived for so
many years.' [*British Medical Journal,* 24 May 1897.]

Thus ended a long conflict and when the President
entertained the Branch at Aldeburgh, Mrs. Newson
Garrett welcomed the doctors in radiant forgetfulness of
the opposition she had shown to her daughter's choice
of a profession thirty years before. Mr. Garrett's death
a few years earlier robbed him of a pleasure which no
one deserved more than he. When in 1885 the Borough
of Aldeburgh received a fresh charter of incorporation
and the bailiffs and burgesses, whose office dated from
Tudor times, were replaced by a mayor, four aldermen
and twelve councillors, Mr. Garrett was elected mayor.
Altogether he served three times: in 1885, 1886 and 1890;
and he gloried in this dignity. But his chief pride was in
his family and perhaps in a special measure in his daughter Elizabeth, on whose behalf he did so much.

12

RETIREMENT

❧

In 1902 Mr. and Mrs. Anderson gave up active work in London and moved to Aldeburgh, where both found new interests. Before following them there, a retrospective glance may be taken at the domestic side of Mrs. Anderson's life while she was in practice. Apart from professional letters she had a large correspondence, writing innumerable family letters which included one to her parents every week; nothing was allowed to interfere with the letter to Alde House on Saturday and bundles of these letters were stored by Mrs. Garrett. They are the affectionate letters of a busy woman: public events jostle with the maladies of the children, usually ascribed to sweets which they managed to get 'on their own hooks'. Her son, especially, was 'very clever' in learning enough of the language even when abroad to buy meringues and cherries. She wrote of the visit of the Shah of Persia, who had a green face; and of Mr. Gladstone at church in the adjoining pew, enunciating the Athanasian Creed with extreme fervour: 'not three incomprehensibles' but 'one incomprehensible'. To the writer, he formed a fourth incomprehensible. Then there was the Dreyfus case and the death of Queen Victoria. Coming to more personal affairs she commented proudly on honours won by the London School of Medicine for Women and donations to the New Hospital. News of the family and any distinctions won by them were referred to: such as the visit of Professor Henry Fawcett, then Postmaster-General, and Mrs. Fawcett to Aberfeldy in 1880, when they attended the Gillies' Ball given by the Prince and Princess of Wales. 'Harry' committed the enormity of shaking hands with Queen Victoria, but possibly she forgave him as he was blind. The distinctions won at Cambridge by Philippa Fawcett in 1890 and a little later by Philip Cowell were subjects for rejoicing. When on holiday abroad Mrs. Anderson described the architecture of Cologne Cathedral and noted the width in feet of the Danube. Her handwriting remained clear and forceful. She wrote with the goose quills of her youth, cutting them herself, and woe betide any one who touched them. She never had a secretary nor a typewriter, but dealt unaided with a mass of correspondence which would have been the despair of most people.

In 1888 the Rev. John Llewelyn Davies accepted a living at Kirby Lonsdale. That he and his wife should leave London for such a distant part of England was a source of regret to Mrs. Anderson, who wrote to their daughter, Margaret:

Retirement

'I cannot refuse you anything just now so "as you are strong, be merciful". I will come on the 2nd as you wish [probably to speak at a meeting]. I am so very very sorry you are all going and I am afraid you will all be sorry too in three months. The publicity of the country is so fatiguing. I am not quite sure that I want to see any of you again before you go. It is worse than twenty funerals.'

A few years later Mrs. Llewelyn Davies died, and in the depth of a particularly cold winter Mrs. Anderson went to the funeral at Kirby Lonsdale.

To her children, especially while they were at school, Mrs. Anderson wrote with unfailing regularity, usually sending two letters a week to each. Short extracts from their replies illustrate their friendship with her. In 1890 Louie was at St. Leonard's [St. Andrews] in the house of the head mistress, Miss Frances Dove, who, as an early Girton student, knew Miss Emily Davies and sometimes invited her to stay at the school-house. The letter refers to one of these visits.

L.G.A. to E.G.A.   *St. Leonard's, 8 June 1890*

'I don't think Miss Davies and Miss Dove seem great friends. They squash each other rather. Miss Davies is dry and snubs Miss Dove's theories to our joy. The other day Miss Dove announced that girls ought not to get letters at school, a short one once a fortnight was more than sufficient to keep them posted in home events. Miss Davies: "I never heard that letters were an evil before." Dove: "They occupy their minds and their attention away from school life." Miss Davies: "I should have thought that they might contain admonition to work."'

The following year Alan was at Eton where he had gained a place in College. The reference is to a photograph of himself and his dog seated on a sofa.

A.G.A. to E.G.A.   *Eton, 17 May 1891*
'I wish Don was seperated [*sic*] from me because I don't like always looking at myself but I do like looking at Don.' Later, 'I have gummed up Don in my room.'

When Mr. Llewelyn Davies died Mrs. Anderson was unable to travel or even to write, but a letter from her sister, Mrs. Fawcett, to Miss Llewelyn Davies expressed the regard both she and Elizabeth felt for him.

M.G.F. to M.Ll.D.   *24 May 1916*
'. . . When I heard of your father's death my mind went back to Elizabeth's early struggle about the medical profession and to Miss Emily Davies' pioneer work for education and I remembered how he had stood for these aspects of the whole woman's movement towards freedom. You must be very proud of his record.'

A very full life and a dominant idea of service have drawbacks. Mrs. Anderson neither had the time nor felt the need, outside her home, for those friendships which spring from close spiritual communion and need leisure. Her relation to her sister Louie was of this character and she gave such an affection to her husband and in later life to her children, but to no one else. Miss Emily Davies was the closest and most important friend of her youth and she never forgot the debt she owed her, but little sentiment entered into Elizabeth's friendship with Emily. Their letters might have passed between two brother officers on active service. She easily established amiable relations which went by the name of friendship. She was not exacting and once her respect was gained, as far as time permitted, she liked 'to make friends' widely, not asking for superior ability or outstanding qualities. To the magic gift of charm—which she did not see in herself—she capitulated at once. Mrs. Russell Gurney possessed this quality in a high degree, and in later life Mrs. Anderson acknowledged it in Mrs. Llewelyn Davies and a few other friends.

Hospitable by inclination, she liked visitors who knew when to leave. 'Will not your mother be anxious if you stay longer?' helped a shy young man to move off promptly. Miss Cock, who followed her as dean of the School, retained a vivid memory of a dinner-party at which the chief guest was a young and diffident bride, and when the golden moment for departure had come and gone, the hostess made an excuse to write a note which she slipped into Miss Cock's hand, 'For goodness sake—Go!'

Retirement

To her nieces, who often stayed with her, she would say at breakfast, giving a sovereign to each: 'There, my dears, you can go where you like and do what you like: don't let me see you again till the evening and remember dinner will be at seven o'clock and you must be home in time to dress.' Then she would take them to a theatre —to a play by Shakespeare from choice, provided that Falstaff were not in it. She insisted that her nephews and nieces should learn to dance and provided lessons and then parties for them. Some she sent to public school and one to college.

In dealing with her own son and daughter she avoided a mistake of many parents. She did not treat them as children when they began to think themselves grown up. With a deference and respect denied to Miss Davies in the past, she accepted their opinions and took their advice. When Alan was about six years old, his mother went to Court. The younger medical women were distinguishing themselves and some took up important work abroad. As the dean of the medical school, she wanted to be able to present them before they left for India. The first step was to choose the material for the court gown. A peach-coloured satin was unrolled. Mrs. Anderson admired it, but before buying turned to her son. 'Much too young,' was his comment and so something more matronly was substituted.

Generally tactful with people, on occasion her honesty was embarrassing. To the visitor who told her that Mr.

Retirement

Gladstone had offered him a seat in his cabinet, she said, thinking aloud: 'Dear me, I knew he was short of good men but I had no idea it was as bad as that.' Extreme frankness also marked the entries in her visitors' book in which she usually but not invariably wrote herself. 'Never want to see her again,' appears against one name.

To the young, she pointed out two classes into which people fall—'getters' and 'givers', making it clear that they should join the latter group. Another division she favoured was 'absorbents' and 'radiants', having no patience with those who spread gloom to others. To the world she appeared a practical, able woman, a little brusque perhaps, and sometimes hard; yet her heart was very tender. The sight of a brakeload of children cheering shrilly and away to the country for a day's outing always brought tears. 'I know it is silly,' she said, 'but I can't help it. They are so happy and it is so little.'

Apart from medicine, she read considerably but could not bear any approach to impropriety. Sargent, the artist, while painting her portrait in 1901 recommended her to read *Thaïs* by Anatole France. He could not praise it too highly—a work of art, etc., so she bought a copy in order to read it during a holiday in Spain. After a few pages its fate was sealed. She tore it into fragments the size of a postage-stamp in order not to demoralize the inhabitants as she scattered it over the arid countryside.

She enjoyed fine stitchery, drawn-thread work especially, and she introduced home industries to Aldeburgh

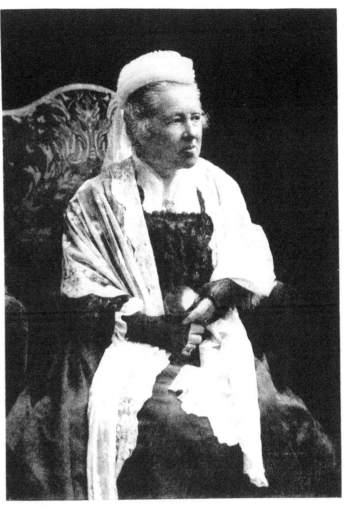

ELIZABETH GARRETT ANDERSON, AGED 73
photograph by Olive Edis, F.R.P.S.
(Mrs. E. H. Galsworthy)

and also encouraged musical taste there by arranging concerts of classical music by good artists. As a girl she had played the piano but she was no musician. Her inability even to whistle accounts for a family story against her. When Alan was at school he could not bear to think that Don, a large black and tan collie, was short of exercise. 'CRUEL,' he said, and as his mother agreed, Don joined the brougham when it took her to visit her patients. His voice was strident and he barked incessantly. Occasionally she went by omnibus and Don followed. One day leaving the bus she forgot Don till, as it rumbled away, she heard his familiar voice in the distance. In distress she turned to a bystander. 'Whistle,' she said, 'please whistle.' 'What am I to whistle for?' 'Never mind that, WHISTLE,' but it was too late: the omnibus, with Don circling round it, was on its way to the Mile End Road. Another humanitarian suggestion made by his master on behalf of Don was that his thirst should be relieved during these drives. 'It would be so easy for you, Mother, to carry a saucer and a flask of water. I think it is a SHAME not to do so.' However, she drew the line at this. All her life she had been a keen gardener. Years ago the garden-labourer had said, 'Mrs. Anderson be a power of help to me,' and in retirement as long as her strength lasted she remained the best member of her outdoor staff.

In 1902 the family circle was enriched by a daughter-in-law, an immense pleasure to Mr. and Mrs. Anderson, who in due course became the proudest of grandparents. On the morning when the first grandson appeared Mr. Anderson informed his friends in the city that it was a magnificent baby, weighing twelve stone! When, as an infant, this grandchild visited them, Mrs. Anderson wrote of him, 'our beloved, the joy of our lives, the sweetest of children'.

In 1907 Mr. Anderson died. A quarter of a century earlier he had started a golf course at Aldeburgh which brought prosperity to the place. He served as captain of the club and as mayor of the borough for years. As chief magistrate he had his own methods of dealing with the turbulent youth of Aldeburgh. Police-inspector Mann brought some boys before the mayor. They had been caught red-handed destroying young trees. 'You must never trouble Inspector Mann like this again. He has his own work to do. Surely you have your own Inspector Mann inside you?' So with a warning and a bun, they were dismissed to wonder how so large a person could fit into their jackets and perhaps, after much thought, to grasp his meaning.

It was during his mayoralty that Mr. Anderson's death took place and Mrs. Anderson was invited to continue his year of office. She was the first woman to hold the office of mayor. The following year it was proposed that she should serve again. The Qualifications for Women Act, recently passed, made women eligible for county and borough councils and for the offices of chairman and mayor. She agreed to stand and at the ceremony her election appeared unanimous. She was placed at the table on which the silver maces lay, marked with Queen Elizabeth's cypher. They lent dignity to the proceedings in the Moot Hall, a sixteenth-century building of considerable charm. Unexpectedly, a counsellor arose: he said he had not voted for Mrs. Anderson; at the same time he had no particular objection to her appointment as mayor; he thought, however, she MUST be made to understand that during the year of office she must not invite Mrs. Pankhurst or ANY ONE OF THAT SORT to her house. The public, including friends, were present. Discomfort was general. When would the tirade end? What else would be said? How would Mrs. Anderson reply? When her turn came, the Mayor glanced at the agenda. 'Gentlemen,' she said, 'our first business is the appointment of aldermen.' That was all, but the rebuke was felt.

It was the great question of Votes for Women which perturbed the objecting councillor. All England was ringing with it at that time. For fifty years there had been a society for the enfranchisement of women, named since 1870, 'The National Union of Women's Suffrage Societies', of which Mrs. Fawcett, Mrs. Anderson's sister Millicent, was president. It had organized petitions and deputations and had held countless meetings sometimes addressed by members of Parliament when 'able to spare the time from their parliamentary duties'. These gentlemen were received with suitable deference and generally advocated patience. The society obtained pledges of support from parliamentary candidates who often forgot them when they reached the House of Commons. Perhaps the National Union had done all that could be done constitutionally to alter the law by those without political power. However, the question had not become practical politics. Passion had faded and the young were not attracted: the subject had grown stale. Then suddenly Mrs. Pankhurst and her daughter Christabel, soon joined by Mr. and Mrs. Pethick Lawrence, made Votes for Women the burning question of the day. The Women's Social and Political Union, founded in 1903, became a political force. The agitation was in full swing and Mrs. Anderson, under the influence of the younger generation, had joined the W.S.P.U. when the incident at the Moot Hall took place. In fact Mrs. Pankhurst had visited her recently in order to address a suffrage meeting in Aldeburgh.

Another story of Mrs. Anderson, as Mayor of Aldeburgh, relates to the proclamation of King George V. The Lord Chancellor's missive reached her at night. Early the following morning she called on the deputy mayor. Blows on the door woke Mr. Hall, at 7 a.m. 'Dear me, Mrs. Anderson,' said he, from the bedroom window. 'You are *very* early!' 'Not at all too early, Mr. Hall,' said the Mayor. 'Surely you know the King is dead and arrangements for the Proclamation must be

made.' This she read a few hours later from the steps
of the Moot Hall.

On official occasions Mrs. Garrett Anderson led the
procession up the Church Hill—preceded by the mace-
bearers. A little old woman, in a black velvet bonnet
with the mayoral chain and robe, an unfurled umbrella
in her hand and wearing stout laced boots, she stepped
out bravely to play her part and maintain the dignity of
her office. The corporation in their robes followed her,
and the lifeboat crew, and the Volunteers and the boy
scouts.

When the War started in August 1914, Mrs. Anderson was beyond the consciousness of tragedy. She had
failed in memory and mind. However, on 14 September
she came to London in order to see her daughter and
Dr. Flora Murray leave, in charge of the first unit of
medical women for service in France. At Victoria station
she heard the roll-call for the corps and saw the equipment which she had helped to provide—tons of lint and
cotton wool, cases of instruments, with drugs and
chloroform in wooden crates marked with the Red
Cross and the superscription 'Women's Hospital Corps'.
That such a service by medical women was possible was
due mainly to her. She stood apart, old, bent and con-
fused. Where were they going? To Russia, perhaps?
Never mind: it was a great adventure and to the leaders
she said: 'My dears, if you go, and if you succeed, you
will put forward the women's cause by thirty years.'

Retirement

The port of old age had been reached: the hurricane of
the War passed her by. During the years that followed
her son and daughter could not leave London often.
Martha, the maid, and nurses tended her. 'Toddy', grey
at the muzzle and rheumatic, walked beside her, still
ready to attack other dogs at sight. Martha would present 'another letter from Mr. Alan'. That it could not be
read, that it fell unopened to the floor, did not matter.
It carried the message it was meant to bring, and, to the
end, his letters gave her great pleasure.

On 17 December 1917 she died and was buried at
Aldeburgh which she loved, beside her parents.

Few people work for one cause from youth until old
age. Elizabeth Garrett did so.

Before her mind clouded, walking hand in hand with
her grandson, she confided in him: 'Colin, I have had a
very happy life,' and he, being a polite child, agreed.
She carried happiness within her and by her work
brought happiness to other women.

> Sunset and evening star,
> And one clear call for me.

In her girlhood Elizabeth heard the call to live and
work, and before the evening star lit her to rest she had
helped to tear down one after another the barriers
which, since the beginning of history, hindered women
from work and progress and light and service.

APPENDIXES

Appendix 1

MISCELLANEOUS

>>⟫⟫■◦◅◅◅

THE GARRETT FAMILY[1]

NEWSON GARRETT   *b.* July 1812
     m. April 1834
     d. May 1893 at 81

LOUISA DUNNELL   *b.* May 1813
     m. April 1834
     d. January 1903 at 90

Their children:

LOUISA MARIA   *b.* 1835
     m. 1857 James William Smith
     d. 1867

ELIZABETH   *b.* 9 June 1836
     m. 9 Feb .1871 J. G. S. Anderson
     d. 17 December 1917

Their children:

     LOUISA GARRETT, *b.* July 1873
     MARGARET SKELTON, *b.* Sept. 1874;
       d. Dec. 1875
     ALAN GARRETT, *b.* March 1877

[1] From a table by Mrs. Herbert Cowell and others.

Miscellaneous

DUNNELL NEWSON	*b.*	1837; *d.* 1838 (6 months)
NEWSON DUNNELL	*b.*	1839; *d.* 1916
EDMUND	*b.*	1840; *d.* 1914
ALICE	*b.*	1842
	m.	1863 Herbert Cowell
	d.	1925
AGNES	*b.*	1845
	d.	1935
MILLICENT	*b.*	1847
	m.	1867 Henry Fawcett
	d.	1929
SAMUEL	*b.*	1850
	d.	1923
JOSEPHINE	*b.*	1853
	m.	1873 Charles Salmon
	d.	1925
GEORGE HERBERT	*b.*	1854
	d.	1929

See Chapter 2.

THE MIDDLESEX HOSPITAL, 1860
MEMBERS OF THE STAFF[1]

MR. WILLIAM HAWES	Governor
MR. THOMAS NUNN	Surgeon & Dean of the Medical School 1859-67

[1] From information furnished by the Middlesex Hospital.

Miscellaneous

MR. CAMPBELL DE MORGAN	Surgeon. Treasurer of the Medical School 1845
DR. STEWART	Physician 1855-66
DR. THOMPSON	Physician 1859-79
DR. JOHN MURRAY	Physician 1871-5
MR. WILLIS	Resident Medical Assistant
MR. WORTHINGTON	House Surgeon
MR. JOSHUA PLASKITT	Apothecary

See Chapter 4.

From the *Spectator*, 8 *November* 1862
NEWS OF THE WEEK

'Miss Garrett's admission to matriculation at St. Andrews is still in doubt, although she has been accepted by the Secretary and given class tickets by two professors. The Senate is to deliberate formally on the question. Her father is to try the case, if necessary, in court, and anyhow the Senate's vote may be favourable as the chance to secure all wealthy female medical students is worth something to a small University.'

From the *Spectator*, 22 *November* 1862
NEWS OF THE WEEK

'. . . legal authorities consulted by Mr. Garrett have decided that an innovation such as the admission of female students is outside the power of any professor,

Miscellaneous

and can only be decided by the Senate. It appears therefore that Scottish as well as English Universities are to be shut to women. Both at Edinburgh and St. Andrews, however, the authorities may be willing to establish separate female medical classes.'

By permission of the Editor of the Spectator.

From the Lancet, 18 June 1870

The Paris Correspondent of the *Lancet* writes 'in haste' to describe 'the medical event of the day'. It is the first time a lady has graduated at the Paris Faculty. Ladies, relatives and friends of Miss Garrett, have been for once admitted into the 'salle des Etats'. Miss Garrett wore 'the traditional gown and bands hitherto reserved on such occasions for the male sex', and 'presented a most pleasing appearance'. Her success was referred to in flattering terms. The hall was 'literally crowded with students', and after the ceremony as Miss Garrett crossed the court 'almost all the students' bowed to their 'lady confrère'. All doctors and judges expressed 'more or less liberal opinions' about lady doctors, M. Broca being especially enthusiastic. The Faculty was really 'en fête' and every one under the influence of such novel and important events.

By permission of the Editor of the Lancet.

See Chapter 5.

Miscellaneous

PRECIS NOTES of MINUTE BOOK of BOARD MEETINGS of EAST LONDON HOSPITAL for CHILDREN, SHADWELL, 1870

15 *Feb.* Mr. Heckford suggests acquiring the services of Miss Garrett.

16 *March.* Mr. Heckford advises taking Miss Garrett as visiting Medical Officer to the Hospital. 'Strike out a new path in expectation of gaining the suffrage of the public.' Dr. Barnes will not commit himself to recommending the employment of a woman doctor, but recommends Miss Garrett on his knowledge of her character. She is finally accepted, due chiefly to Mr. Heckford's influence in her favour.

23 *March.* Miss Garrett has joined the staff.

21 *June.* Miss Garrett and Mrs. Heckford made visiting officers of the Hospital for a month.

23 *August.* Miss Garrett concerns herself with the management of the Out-Patient Department.

30 *August.* Miss Garrett in spite of some opposition from the Committee arranges that a sub-committee is formed to deal with the management of the Out-Patient Department.

11 *October.* Miss Garrett admits a patient with dropsy plus scarlatina; censured by Committee.

See Chapter 5.

Miscellaneous

From *Punch*, 26 *November* 1870

A first-page article headed 'Vote for the Ladies' describes the work of the future School Board and the candidature of Miss Garrett, M.D., for Marylebone.

'As to Miss Garrett, who, to her long practical acquaintance with the above things, adds sound medical knowledge, and can advise on all sanatory questions connected with schools, she will be an invaluable acquisition to the Board; and Marylebone should be proud that the richest and most educated of the districts can send to that Council one who will render such services. Miss Garrett and the other ladies profess no "strong-minded women's" doctrines, but those which all rational men would teach.'

From *Punch*, 10 *December* 1870

From a comment headed 'Our Educationists': 'Well done, gallant Greenwich and gallanter Marylebone! Your chivalry will be rewarded: Emily Davies and Elizabeth Garrett will not be the least useful members of the new Council.'

And again: 'We have been electing a School-Board— London has chosen her men and women. Two of the latter have got in, and I do not see why they should not prove the best members. One of them, a delightful lady, a friend of mine, and a Doctor of Medicine, headed everybody by a terrific majority.'

By permission of the Proprietors of *Punch*.

See Chapter 6.

Miscellaneous

THE WOMEN who MATRICULATED at
EDINBURGH, 1869, were:

Miss Sophia Jex-Blake
Mrs. Isabel Thorne
Miss Edith Pechey (Mrs. Pechey Phipson)
Mrs. Evans
Miss Chaplin (Mrs. Chaplin Ayrton)
Miss Mary Anderson (Mrs. Marshall)
Miss Bovell

THE SONG OF THE WOMEN
(from *Departmental Ditties*, 1929 edition)

Eight stanzas express the gratitude of Indian women
to Lady Dufferin. Their message of love and thankful-
ness is to go across the world. Stanzas 4, 6, and 7, dealing
with their need of medical aid, are quoted in full.

By Life that ebbed with none to staunch the failing,
  By Love's sad harvest garnered ere the spring,
When Love in Ignorance wept unavailing
O'er young buds dead before their blossoming;
    By all the grey owl watched, the pale moon viewed,
    In past grim years declare our gratitude!

If she have sent her servants in our pain,
  If she have fought with Death and dulled his sword;
If she have given back our sick again,

Miscellaneous

And to the breast the weakling lips restored,
Is it a little thing that she has wrought?
Then Life and Death and Motherhood be naught.

Go forth, O wind, our message on thy wings,
And they shall hear thee pass and bid thee speed,
In reed-roofed hut, on white-walled home of kings
Who have been holpen by her in their need.
All spring shall give thee fragrance, and the wheat
Shall be a tasselled floorcloth to thy feet.

(By kind permission of Mrs. Rudyard Kipling and
Messrs. Methuen & Co.)
See Chapter 9.

IN MAY 1878 NINE WOMEN WERE ON THE MEDICAL REGISTER

The names are given in the order of registration

Elizabeth Blackwell	1858
Elizabeth Garrett Anderson	1865
Eliza Walker Dunbar	1877
Frances Hoggan	
Sophia Jex-Blake	
Louisa Atkins	
Edith Pechey	
Annie R. Barker	1878
Ann E. Clark	

See Chapter 9.

Miscellaneous

IN 1887 FIFTY-EIGHT WOMEN WERE ON THE MEDICAL REGISTER

NUMBER OF STUDENTS AT THE LONDON SCHOOL OF MEDICINE FOR WOMEN

1887 77 Students
1889 91 Students, fees covered expenses
1892 133 Students, heavy deficit owing to building and repairs
1896 159 Students and an unprecedented entry of 50 new Students
1903 318 Students
1917 441 Students

Appendix 2

BIOGRAPHICAL NOTES

>>>⇒●⇐<<

Adams, Professor J. C., 1819–92
  Early studied astronomy. Senior wrangler and first Smith's prizeman 1843. Concerned in discovery of planet Neptune. One of the first members of Girton College appointed by the Senate 1880. His calculations concerning planet Neptune were suggested by a passage in *The Connection of the Physical Sciences* by Mary Somerville.
D.N.B.
Emily Davies and Girton College by Barbara Stephen

Amberley, John Russell, Viscount Amberley, 1842–76
  Eldest son Lord John [later Earl] Russell shocked society by free thought, feminism and advocacy of birth-control.

D.N.B.
The Amberley Papers

Amberley, Lady Katharine Louisa Stanley, 1842–74
  M. 1864 John Russell Viscount Amberley. Influenced by J. S. Mill, friend George Eliot, Elizabeth Garrett,

Biographical Notes

Emily Davies. Ardent feminist: spoke at woman suffrage meetings. Helped entry women into medical profession. Caught diphtheria from her child and died age 32.

The Amberley Papers

Barnett, the Rev. [later Canon] Samuel Augustus, 1844-1913
Social reformer, principally remembered for work in Whitechapel, where he was responsible, among other things, for the formation of the Whitechapel Art Gallery. Friend of Octavia Hill and a prime mover in the foundation of the Charity Organization Society. Founder of the University Settlement movement and first warden of Toynbee Hall. A member of Elizabeth Garrett's election committee for first London School Board.

D.N.B.

Blackwell, Elizabeth, 1821-1910
Born at Bristol, emigrated U.S.A. Started school for girls in Cincinnati. Studied medicine privately while teaching. After many difficulties graduated M.D. Geneva, U.S.A., 1849. Lost sight one eye, returned to London and admitted automatically to British Medical Register 1858. Lectured in London on Medicine as a Profession for Ladies: influenced Elizabeth Garrett. Returned to America and founded hospital for women in New York, at which Sophia Jex-Blake was an early student.

D.N.B.

Biographical Notes

Bodichon, Barbara Leigh Smith, 1827-91

Eldest d. Benjamin Smith, M.P. Norwich. Knew anti-corn law politicians: took great interest in all questions relating to education and general improvement in the position of women. Much interested in wrongs of Caroline Norton and wrote brief and lucid pamphlet on laws relating to women 1854 which helped to procure passage of Equal Custody of Infants Act. 1857 m. Dr. Bodichon of Algiers. Friend of George Eliot, Miss Parkes (later Mme Belloc) with whom responsible 1858 for establishing the *Englishwomen's Journal,* which led directly to the formation of the Society for the Employment of Women. Influenced Emily Davies towards women's movement and collaborated with her in first plan of Girton College. Water-colour artist and benefactress to Hitchin and Girton College and also to Bedford College for Women. Supported Elizabeth Garrett.

D.N.B.

Emily Davies and Girton College, by Barbara Stephen

Butler, Josephine, 1828-1906

D. John Grey of Dilston: m. Rev. George Butler 1852. After marriage lived at Oxford, Cheltenham, Liverpool and Winchester, where her husband held educational or ecclesiastical appointments. From youth devoted herself to moral elevation of women, receiving whole-hearted support from her husband. 1869 engaged in agitation for repeal of Contagious Diseases Acts of 1864, 1866 and 1869. Hon. Secretary of the Ladies' National Association for Repeal, formed 1869. For 16 years Mrs. Butler was indefatigable in cause: secured important political victory in 1870 when at by-election in Colchester the Government candidate Sir Henry Storks, who championed the Acts, was defeated by propaganda against them. In H. of C. Sir James Stansfeld [see Stansfeld] led opposition to Acts. In 1883 Acts partially and in 1886 totally repealed.

D.N.B.
Josephine Butler,
published by Ass. Moral & Social Hygiene

Cobbe, Frances Power, 1822-1904

Was attracted to the women's movement by Mary Carpenter. In 1862 read before the Social Science Congress a paper on the admission of women to university degrees. Her chief interests seem to have been the anti-vivisection and the philanthropical movements, but she also supported the cause of woman suffrage and took great interest in Girton College.

D.N.B.

Courtney, Leonard Henry, first Baron Courtney of Penwith,
1832-1918

Journalist and statesman. In 1865 leader-writer to *The Times* under John Delane, also contributed to the *Fortnightly Review*. Entered Parliament in 1875 as liberal member for Liskeard: collaborated with Henry Fawcett, Joseph Chamberlain and Sir Charles Dilke. Perhaps the greatest British statesman since Cobden of those who have not held Cabinet rank.

Persistently advocated tolerance and conciliation during S. African War. Deeply opposed to Great War. Staunch supporter of women's movement.

D.N.B.

Crabbe, George, 1754-1832

Born at Aldeburgh, Suffolk, father 'saltmaster' of the town. Was apprenticed to various surgeons, set up in practice independently but unsuccessful, and in 1780 came to London to try his fortune in literature. After repeated losses applied successfully for the patronage of Burke, who advised him to take orders and he became chaplain to the Duke and Duchess of Rutland 1782. Scott, Wordsworth, Jane Austen and E. Fitzgerald are all quoted as admirers of his works, of which *The Village*, i.e. Aldeburgh (1783), is one.

D.N.B.

Davies, Rev. John Llewelyn, 1826-1916

Fourth son of Rev. John Davies, D.D., Rector of Gateshead. President of Union Society at Cambridge, as an undergraduate known for interest in politics and social questions. All his life supported the movement for higher education for women, in which his sister Emily Davies played so important a part. Ordained 1851.

Biographical Notes

Appointed to rectory of Christ Church, Marylebone. In 1873-4 and 1878-86 was principal of Queen's College, Harley Street, supported the women's suffrage movement and that for the extension to women of university degrees. Much influenced by Rev. F. D. Maurice. Personal friend to Elizabeth Garrett: served on her Election Committee for London School Board, as member of managing committee of New Hospital for Women and as member of the council of the London School of Medicine for Women.

D.N.B.

Emily Davies and Girton College, by Barbara Stephen

Davies, Sarah Emily, 1830-1921

Through her brother, Rev. J. Llewelyn Davies, Rector Christ Church, Marylebone, was able to do some work for the *Englishwomen's Journal* (founded 1858 by Mme Bodichon and Miss Parkes, later Mme Belloc) and for the Society for Promoting the Employment of Women. After her father's death in 1860, Miss Davies came to London and in 1862 became honorary secretary of a committee for the admission of women to university examinations. [This committee was instituted largely owing to Elizabeth Garrett's experiences in trying to obtain a medical education and degree.] Influenced and helped Elizabeth Garrett enormously.

In 1865 Miss Davies' committee secured the admission of girls to the Cambridge local examinations and in 1866 she founded the London Schoolmistresses' Association. In 1864 a memorial for which she was responsible caused girls' schools to be included in the scope of the Schools Inquiry Commission (1864-8), before which she gave evidence. In 1867 Miss Davies began to organize a college for women, of which Hitchin (1869) and Girton (1873) were the result. From 1873 Girton College, of which she was the first mistress, its finances, students and relations with the University of Cambridge became Miss Davies' chief interest.

Miss Davies also took an important part in the women's suffrage question. Helped Mme Bodichon and Miss Parkes to organize a petition to Parliament (presented by J. S. Mill) in 1866. In 1904 when she resigned the honorary secretaryship of Girton College became Chairman of the London Society for Women's Suffrage.

Emily Davies and Girton College, by Barbara Stephen

Faithfull, Emily

April 1862, manager of the Victoria Women's Printing Press, started by the Society for Promoting the Employment of Women.

Fawcett, Henry, 1833-84

Born at Salisbury, son of William Fawcett, draper and mayor, afterwards farmer. Early determined to enter Parliament in order to forward education and improve conditions of farm labourers. Educated at King's Col-

Biographical Notes

lege School, London, Peterhouse, Cambridge (1852), and Trinity Hall (1853). Lost his sight (1858) as result of accident but returned to Trinity Hall of which he was a Fellow, and continued to study political economy. Disciple and friend of J. S. Mill. Elected Professor of Political Economy Cambridge 1863. M. Millicent Garrett 1867, lived in Cambridge during term, in London for parliamentary session. Liberal M.P. for Brighton 1865, and for Hackney 1874. Throughout life, ardent and wise supporter of women's movement. Acted as teller for J. S. Mill in debate for inclusion of women in extension of parliamentary franchise, 1867. Helped movement for medical education of women. Appointed Postmaster-General 1880, though without a seat in Cabinet. As P.M.G. introduced many reforms—6d. telegrams, parcel post, etc., and improved pay and conditions for staff and facilitated the employment of women in the Post Office. Appointed first medical woman in P.O. to attend women employees. Popularly known in H. of C. as 'member for Hindustan', owing to his interest in India and concern for just treatment of native peoples.

One of the founders of Newnham College.

Constant supporter of medical women.

D.N.B.
Chambers's Encyclopaedia
Private information

Biographical Notes

Fawcett, Dame Millicent Garrett, G.B.E., LL.D., J.P. (Mrs. Henry Fawcett), 1847-1929

Daughter of Newson and Louisa Garrett. Influenced in youth by her elder sister Elizabeth, whose efforts to enter medical profession predisposed her to support women's movement. Married 1867 Henry Fawcett, Professor Economics Cambridge, and M.P. Brighton. Through husband met J. S. Mill and other radical thinkers. In 1869 the lecture movement which resulted in the foundation of Newnham College was launched from her house. In 1870 published *Political Economy for Beginners*. Made her first public speech for enfranchisement of women in 1868 and to the end of her life made this cause her chief aim. President National Union for Women's Suffrage Societies for many years. By her leadership and wise advocacy of the claims of women to the parliamentary vote foundation was laid to the success of the movement in 1918. In Westminster Abbey there is a memorial to Henry Fawcett and to his wife.

The Cause by R. Strachey
What I Remember, by M. G. Fawcett
D.N.B.

Grote, George, 1794-1871

Educated at Charterhouse, went into the family banking business, studied classics, political economy and philosophy. Married 1820 Harriet Lewin, and became friendly with James Mill and Bentham. Keenly inter-

Biographical Notes

ested in the project for a University of London, and with Brougham, Mill and Thomas Campbell was one of the founders. A dispute as to the professor of moral philosophy (Grote was determined that the appointee should not be a minister of any religion) led to Grote's withdrawal (1830). He entered parliament (1832) as Liberal member for the City of London, and remained till 1841; during his parliamentary career he advocated voting by ballot, but was not successful. In 1845 he resigned his position at the bank, and devoted himself fully to *History of Greece* begun before he entered parliament. Member of the Senate of the University of London in 1850, active in procuring the new charter of 1858 and became Vice-Chancellor in 1861. From that year until 1868 he endeavoured to get women admitted to the examinations. Supported efforts of women to enter medical profession and to obtain good general education.

D.N.B.

Grote, Harriet, 1792–1878

Daughter of a Madras civil servant. Biographer, talented hostess and musician, the brilliant wife of George Grote. Befriended Jenny Lind and cultivated the friendship of Mendelssohn, as well as keeping open house for her husband's Radical-reformer friends while he was in Parliament. Had numerous friends among the public men of France, especially Comte. Advocate of parliamentary enfranchisement of women, admission of women on equal terms with men to the University of London examinations and to the medical profession.

D.N.B.

Gurney, Rt. Hon. Russell, M.P., 1804-78

Son of Sir John Gurney, Baron of the Exchequer. Educated at Trinity College, Cambridge. Called to the Bar at the Inner Temple in 1828. Common Pleader in the City of London 1830-45 (when he became Q.C.). In 1850 appointed judge of Sheriffs' Court and in 1856 Common Sergeant. He became Recorder in 1857, M.P. (Conservative) for Southampton in 1865. As M.P. had charge of several important Acts, including the Married Women's Property Act 1870 and Medical Act 1876 which gave permissive power to the medical examining bodies in the U.K. to admit women to their qualifying examinations. He married 1852 Emelia Batten. Mrs. Russell Gurney born 1823, died 1896, was a friend of Emily Davies and Elizabeth Garrett, helped to secure a medical education for Miss Garrett, and was a member of Girton College 1872-96 and promoter of New Hospital for Women and London School of Medicine for Women.

D.N.B.

The Hon. Mr. Justice Hannen
Sir James, Baron Hannen (life peer), 1821-94

In 1870, Hannen was a judge of the Court of Queen's

Biographical Notes

Bench, and a sergeant-at-law, and had been knighted (in 1868).

D.N.B.

Haweis, the Rev. Hugh Reginald, 1838-1901

Musician, author and popular preacher. Incumbent (1866) of St. James's, Westmoreland Street, Marylebone, where his 'popular services and spectacular appearances in the pulpit combined to fill the church till he died. He was interested in the provision of open spaces in London, in Sunday opening of museums and picture galleries, and through his wife, Mary, daughter of Thomas Musgrave Joy, the artist, in women's suffrage. Mary Haweis published in 1897 a novel called *A Flame of Fire* to vindicate the helplessness of womenkind.'

D.N.B.

Hill, Octavia, 1838-1912

Her name is chiefly connected with improvements in housing conditions for the very poor, and her importance to the women's movement rests primarily on her successful management of a business concern in which she relied on women helpers trained by herself. John Ruskin first supplied some capital for purchase of tenement houses and in management of these her work began in 1864. She opened up a new career to women, and at the same time carried out a far-reaching social reform in housing conditions. At her death Octavia Hill was in charge of 2,000 tenancies. Was ardent advocate of pre-

Biographical Notes

servation of open spaces, university settlements, cadet movement, and other forms of corporate social work among London poor. Supporter of Charity Organization Society. Believed in private enterprise; could not have foreseen developments in rate-aided housing and social services. Her work led to foundation of National Trust, 1895. Her personality and appearance must have been striking and most attractive.

D.N.B.
Society of Women Housing Managers,
13 Suffolk St., S.W.1.

Hughes, Thomas, 1822-96
Educated Rugby under Dr. Arnold—and Oriel College, Oxford. Barrister. Q.C. 1869. Disciple Rev. F. D. Maurice and helped him to found Working Men's College, being principal 1872-83. Published anonymously *Tom Brown's School Days,* 1857.

D.N.B.

Huxley, Professor T. H., 1825-95
Born at Ealing of schoolmaster parentage. Not formally educated after the age of eight, but widely read and always interested in scientific subjects. Became apprentice to a doctor brother-in-law in 1841, obtained a scholarship to Charing Cross Hospital in 1842. Accompanied a surveying voyage to Australia 1846-50, as assistant surgeon. Taught at the Royal School of Mines.

Biographical Notes

Closely associated with the controversies excited by the publication, 1859, of Darwin's *Origin of Species*. Applied the methods of Descartes to the study of science, i.e. he 'held doubt to be a duty'. He was a member of the first School Board for London (1870) and wrote an essay on its duties (*Contemporary Review* 1870). He left the Board in 1872. He supported the parliamentary enfranchisement of women and the medical education of women. He was an original governor of the London School of Medicine for Women (1875).

D.N.B.

Jex-Blake, Sophia, 1840–1912

Entered Queen's College, London, 1858 as student and 1859 became mathematical tutor. In 1865 she went to U.S.A. and studied (1868) in Dr. Elizabeth Blackwell's Hospital, New York. In 1868 on death of her father returned to England, where she found insuperable difficulty in continuing her medical studies. Finally, she and six other women were permitted to matriculate in Faculty Medicine, Edinburgh University, 1869. Professors in medicine refused to teach women. Litigation followed. In 1872 position in Edinburgh hopeless and Miss Jex-Blake came to London. Founded (1874) the London School of Medicine for Women. This almost failed for want of clinical teaching for its students and refusal of all 19 Medical Examining boards in U.K. to accept female candidates. Russell Gurney Enabling Act,

1876, gave these bodies permissive power to examine women and through King & Queen's College of Physicians, Ireland, women obtained registrable licences. Miss Jex-Blake introduced Sir James Stansfeld, M.P., to London School of Medicine for Women and persuaded him to become hon. treasurer. He collaborated with chairman, Royal Free Hospital, and obtained facilities for clinical teaching of the women students there.

Miss Jex-Blake, already M.D. Berne [not registrable degree, as it was a foreign one], obtained legal qualification in 1877. In 1878 left London for Edinburgh where she had a private practice and founded a hospital for women 1885, and a school of medicine for women 1886. In 1894 University of Edinburgh admitted women to graduate in Medicine.

Life of Sophia Jex-Blake,
by Dr. Margaret Todd

Leveson-Gower, Granville George, second Earl Granville,
    1815-91
Had a long public career, both in foreign and colonial affairs. Was Chancellor of London University from 1856-91.

Lind, Jenny, 1820-87
Johanna Maria Lind, later known as Madame Jenny Lind-Goldschmidt.

Born at Stockholm 1820; became a British subject by the naturalization of her husband, the composer Otto

Biographical Notes

Goldschmidt, in 1859. Died at Malvern 1887. Was a personal friend of Mendelssohn and of Harriet Grote. Among her interests were the Bach Choir, founded 1876, whose women members she trained and superintended, and the Royal College of Music, where she was chief Professor of Singing from 1883-6.

D.N.B.

Lockyer, Joseph Norman, 1836-1920

Son of a Rugby physician. Became a clerk in the War Office, studying astronomy in his spare time. By 1870 acquired the reputation of a good government servant and administrator, and a first-rate scientist. Was transferred to the Science and Art Department at South Kensington (1875); had been secretary to the Royal Commission on Scientific Instruction. Started the Science Museum at South Kensington and was made first professor of astronomical physics at the new Royal College of Science. From early manhood a friend of J. G. S. Anderson and in sympathy with the women's movement.

D.N.B.

Loftie, William John, 1839-1911

Graduated from Trinity College, Dublin, in 1862. Took holy orders 1865, and was curate at St. James's, Westmoreland Street, 1869-71. He was assistant chaplain at the Chapel Royal, Savoy, till 1895. His chief interest was in London antiquities, but he wrote fre-

Biographical Notes

quently in the *People's Magazine,* the *Guardian,* the *Saturday Review,* and other papers.

Masson, David, 1822-1907

Professor of Rhetoric and English Literature at Edinburgh University. He had been educated at Aberdeen and earned a living with Chambers, publishers, and through writing for various magazines. He was a friend of Carlyle and his wife. While at Edinburgh he interested himself in the movement for women's education and until the admission of women to the Scottish universities gave annually (from 1868) a course of lectures to women on English literature. These were under the auspices of the Association for the University Education of Women. Friend of Elizabeth Garrett and Sophia Jex-Blake, introducing the latter to Rt. Hon. James Stansfeld, M.P.

D.N.B.

Maurice, the Rev. F. D.

The only son of eight children of a Unitarian preacher. Greatly influenced throughout life by his sisters and became promoter of better education for women about whom he held unusually broad-minded views. Studied law. Went to Cambridge University but could not take degree as unable to make subscriptions then necessary. In 1831 baptized as member of C. of E.; ordained 1834; Chaplain to Guy's Hospital 1836; Chaplain, Lincoln's Inn Fields 1846. Founded Queen's College for Women

Biographical Notes

with help of other professors at King's College 1848. Always ardent advocate for education of women but opposed to the study of biology by them and still more to women studying medicine or entering any of the learned professions. Character said to have been most fascinating. Kingsley called him 'the most beautiful human soul' he had known—quite unworldly and very broad-minded in theology and in question of women's advancement. One of the first of the clergy to take a prominent part in social movements of his time. Founder and first Principal of Working Men's College. At St. Peter's, Vere Street, London, where he preached 1860-9, he had a large and devoted following.

Life of F. D. Maurice
by his son, General Sir J. F. Maurice, K.C.B.
D.N.B.

Mōhl, Professor, 1800-76

The husband of Mary, *née* Clarke (1793-1883). He was an orientalist, she is described by the D.N.B. as a 'conversationalist' and as having been a friend of Madame Récamier. She was a friend of many distinguished French *littérateurs,* including de Tocqueville, Thiers, Guizot, the Duc de Broglie, etc.

D.N.B.

Norton, Hon. Mrs. Caroline, 1808-77

Granddaughter R. B. Sheridan (1751-1816), witty and beautiful, m. 1827 Hon. George Norton. Three sons were born. Marriage unhappy. In 1836 husband brought civil suit for damages against Lord Melbourne (at that time first step on part of a husband in divorce action), case dismissed. Mrs. Norton's troubles won wide publicity and called attention to the plight under English law of a married woman separated from her husband. His rights in the children were absolute: any money she inherited or earned was his. She could not instruct counsel or institute legal proceedings. She determined to alter the law of England in regard to the economic position of married women and their rights over their children. Caroline Norton's case was of immense importance to the women's movement; she started the agitation which led to the Equal Custody of Infants Act and to the Married Women's Property Act.

The Cause by Ray Strachey
D.N.B.

Procter, Adelaide Ann, 1825-64

Daughter of Bryan Walter Procter, the poet. Educated in literary surroundings. Contributed first poems to the *Book of Beauty* in 1843, and to *Household Words* under the pen name of Mary Berwick from 1853. In 1859 appointed by the Council of the National Association for the Promotion of Social Science to a committee for furthering the employment of women. She edited a volume of verse set up by the women compositors of Miss Emily Faithfull's printing press (itself a venture of

Biographical Notes

the Society for Promoting the Employment of Women).
Miss Procter was interested in all social questions affect-
ing women.

D.N.B.

Russell, Lord John, first Earl Russell, 1792-1878
Third son of 6th Duke of Bedford, K.G. Helped to
frame first Reform Bill passed June 1832. Prime Minister 1846 and again on death of Palmerston in 1865.
Eldest son John Russell Viscount Amberley and his
wife active feminists.

Chambers's Encyclopaedia

*Shaftesbury, Anthony Ashley Cooper, seventh Earl of,
1801-85*
The outstanding philanthropist of the nineteenth century, as Lord Ashley was in House of Commons 1826
until 1851 when he succeeded his father as Earl. His
reforms included more humane treatment for lunatics;
acted as chairman of Lunacy Commission for 56 years,
suppression of the use of boy chimney-sweeps, reform
of conditions of work amongst women and children in
mines and factories. He joined the Ragged School
movement. Supported women's movement, notably
the London School of Medicine for Women and the
New Hospital for Women.

Life of Lord Shaftesbury,
by J. L. Hammond and Barbara Hammond

Biographical Notes

Sidgwick, Henry, 1838-1900

Lecturer in moral philosophy at Cambridge in 1869, when he started lecture scheme for women students, in preparation for local examinations which resulted in the foundation of Newnham College. Sidgwick made himself responsible for the rent of a hall for women students, of which Miss Anne Jemima Clough was superintendent. In 1874 this scheme was superseded by a company and in 1876 Newnham Hall was opened. In 1880 Mrs. Sidgwick (Eleanor Mildred, sister of A. J. Balfour) became Vice-Principal and in 1892 Principal of Newnham and the Sidgwicks lived there till Mr. Sidgwick's death in 1900.

Sidgwick advocated the admission of women to university examinations in 1881, and his retirement from the council of the Senate in 1898 was due partly to the refusal to grant titular degrees to women.

D.N.B.

Simpson, Sir James Young, 1811-70

In 1839 became Professor of Midwifery in Edinburgh University. In 1847 demonstrated that chloroform could be used successfully as an anaesthetic.

Miss Jex-Blake, writing to *The Times* in 1873 (4 September), declared that his death was a great and unexpected blow to the cause of women's medical education at Edinburgh. He had consented to instruct women; had shown himself interested in their studies and would have championed them in the University.

D.N.B.

Biographical Notes

Somerville, Mary, 1780-1872

Daughter of Vice-Admiral Sir. W. G. Fairfax. Famous writer on science and friend of Brougham, Melbourne, Macaulay, etc. Her knowledge of science seems to have been acquired through private reading and the bent of her genius decided by early open-air nature study. The D.N.B. emphasizes her 'feminine charm' as well as her 'masculine breadth of intellect'!

D.N.B.

Stanley, Arthur Penrhyn, 1815-81

Educated Rugby under Dr. Arnold whose life he wrote, and Balliol, Oxford having Tait [afterwards Archbishop of Canterbury] for tutor. 1839 ordained. 1856 Professor of Eccles. Hist. and Canon Christ Church. 1863 Dean of Westminster; accompanied Prince of Wales on earlier tour 1862. Married Lady Augusta Bruce 1863.

Letters of Lady Augusta Stanley
Life of Dean Stanley
D.N.B.

Stanley, Henrietta Maria, Lady Stanley of Alderley, 1807-1895

Daughter 13th Viscount Dillon; married Edward, 2nd Lord Stanley of Alderley.

An outspoken, able, autocratic woman. As Dowager Lady Stanley of Alderley was a great figure in mid-Victorian society and supported foundation of Girton

309

Biographical Notes

College, Queen's College, High Schools for Girls and the London School of Medicine for Women.

The Amberley Papers

Stansfeld, Rt. Hon. James, 1820–98

M.P. Halifax 1859–95. Junior Lord Admiralty 1871–4. Cabinet Minister as President Poor Law Board and President Local Government Board. Friend of Garibaldi who selected Stansfeld as his adviser when he visited England 1864. Sacrificed political career in order to oppose Contagious Diseases Acts introduced into England 1864. Acts repealed 1886, owing mainly to Stansfeld in House of Commons and Mrs. Josephine Butler in constituencies. Stansfeld's interest in disabilities of women began in 1840. He attended anti-slavery convention at Birmingham in June 1840. The convention had been summoned by the British & Foreign Anti-Slavery Society; some 500 delegates attended in response to the invitation addressed to the 'opponents of slavery from every nation and from every clime'. The convention declared that women delegates would not be admitted to the conference. There were about 20 women delegates from U.S.A., all people of standing. Stansfeld was profoundly affected by the event. 'It was that episode and the shame I felt as a man and an Englishman that first turned my thoughts to the position created in England for our mothers, sisters and wives, made me resolve that all schemes of education, of political reform, should include them as equals.' Spoke in London 1869 at the first public meeting for women's suffrage with J. S. Mill, Charles Kingsley, Professor and Mrs. Fawcett, John Morley, Sir Charles Dilke, etc. Through Professor and Mrs. Masson of Edinburgh made acquaintance of Sophia Jex-Blake in 1871 and became interested in efforts of women to enter medical profession. Became hon. treasurer London School of Medicine for Women 1874 and with co-operation of Mr. James Hopgood, chairman of Board of Royal Free Hospital, arranged that clinical instruction should be given to the women students.

Life of James Stansfeld,
by J. L. and Barbara Hammond
Life of Sophia Jex-Blake, by Dr. Margaret Todd

Trelawny, Edward John, 1792-1881

Served in the Royal Navy, had many adventures (according to the autobiographical *Adventures of a Younger Son,* which is not, however, accurate on all points) in the Far East, returned to England 1813 and sought out Shelley in Italy 1821. He was at Leghorn and among Shelley's circle when Shelley was drowned, and was responsible for his funeral arrangements and for sending his wife home to England.

D.N.B.

BIBLIOGRAPHY

A Vindication of the Rights of Women, by Mary Wollstone-
craft.
Life of Mrs. Norton, by J. G. Perkins.
The Cause, by Mrs. Oliver Strachey.
The Life of Florence Nightingale, by Sir Edward Cook.
Florence Nightingale, 1820-56, by I. B. O'Malley.
From One Century to Another, by E. S. Haldane.
The Garretts of Suffolk, a pamphlet by Vincent B. Red-
stone, Fellow of the Royal Historical Society.
Historical and Miscellaneous Questions, by Richmal Mang-
nall.
What I Remember, by Millicent Garrett Fawcett.
Emily Davies and Girton College, by Barbara Stephen.
*Pioneer Work in Opening the Profession of Medicine to
Women*, by Dr. E. Blackwell.
The London School of Medicine for Women, by Mrs. Isabel
Thorne.
The Story of the Middlesex Hospital Medical School, by H.
Campbell Thomson, M.D., F.R.C.P.

Bibliography

Life of Sophia Jex-Blake, by Dr. Margaret Todd.

Life of F. D. Maurice, by his son (Sir J. F. Maurice, K.C.B.).

The Life of Pasteur, by R. Vallory-Radot.

Autobiography of J. S. Mill.

The Subjection of Women, by J. S. Mill.

The Amberley Papers, Ed. by Bertrand and Patricia Russell. Hogarth Press.

Elizabeth Garrett Anderson, an unpublished pamphlet by J. Ford Anderson, M.D.

Jane Austen and Some Contemporaries, by Mona Wilson.

Reminiscences of Mary Scharlieb.

Life of Lord Shaftesbury, by J. L. Hammond and Barbara Hammond.

Life of James Stansfeld, a Victorian Champion of Sex Equality, by J. L. Hammond and Barbara Hammond.

Reports and Minute Books, East London Hospital for Children, Shadwell.

Reports and Minute Books, London (R.F.H.) School of Medicine for Women.

Reports and Minute Books, New Hospital for Women.

British Medical Journal.

Lancet.

The Times.

Punch.

The Spectator.

Dictionary of National Biography, published by the Oxford University Press.

INDEX

>>>>⊃●⋐<<<

A Vindication of the Rights of Women, alluded to, 17

Aberdare, Lord, 221, 222

Aberdeen, an unpleasant reply from a doctor of, 108, 109; Rev. Alexander Anderson at, 145; the University of, 145

Aberfeldy, the Gillies' Ball (1880) at, 265

Academy for Daughters of Gentlemen (Blackheath), The, Elizabeth Garrett at, 32, 33; alluded to, 39

Acton (Middlesex), 63, 64, 85, 179, 180

Adams, Professor J. C., supports Elizabeth Garrett's candidature for School Board, 147; a biographical note of, *app.* 287

Albert (Consort), Prince, Elizabeth Garrett's early recollection of, 26; instals bathroom at Windsor Castle, 33; organizes the Great Exhibition in Hyde Park, *ib.*

Alde House, the Garrett sisters at, 34; alluded to, 36, 264; Elizabeth Garrett at, 36, 37; Elizabeth Gar-

rett leaves, 38; Dr. Elizabeth Blackwell and, 42; Emily Davies visits, 47, 48; a reminiscence of Elizabeth Garrett and Emily Davies at, 48, 49; and Elizabeth Garrett's engagement, 165; Mr. Anderson's reception at, 166

Alde River, The, Newson Garrett's business activities on, 30

Aldeburgh, described, 26; the Garrett's home and life at, 26-9; Newson Garrett's business in, 29, 30; Alde House (*vide*); wrecks in the bay of, 36; the schoolmaster at, 44; letters of Elizabeth Garrett from, 45, 46, 51, 57, 58, 86, 87, 88, 118, 167; Elizabeth Garrett spends Christmas at, 74; alluded to, 76, 86, 108, 202; Elizabeth Garrett's serenity and hopefulness while at, 90; Elizabeth Garrett's studies at, 92; J. G. S. Anderson at, 162, 166; Elizabeth Garrett Anderson removes to, 239; the British Medical Association branch at, 263; Newson Garrett mayor of, *ib.*; Elizabeth Garrett Anderson

315

Index

retires from practice to, 264 *et seq.*; Elizabeth Garrett Anderson introduces home industries to, 270; Elizabeth Garrett Anderson succeeds as Mayor of, 274, 275; a Votes for Women incident at, 273, 274, 275; the Moot Hall at, 273; reminiscences of Elizabeth Garrett Anderson as Mayor of, 274, 275; Elizabeth Garrett Anderson's death at, 276

Alderton (gardener), 35

Alford, Mrs., 121

Algiers, 41

Amberley, Viscount, alluded to, 124, 135, 160; a biographical note of, *app.* 287

Amberley, Viscountess, alluded to, 10, 207; *The Amberley Papers* (*Diary*), 122, 123, 134, 135, 160, 207; a biographical note of, *app.* 287

America, 51, 207, 245

Anderson, Alan Garrett, alluded to, 192 *n.*, 194, 202, 204, 269; birth of, 201; as Chairman of New Hospital for Women, 250; at Eton, 267; the dog of, 271

Anderson, Rev. Alexander, and the Great Disruption of 1843, 144, 145; the household of, 144, 145; and Elizabeth Garrett's notoriety, 165; Elizabeth Garrett sends photos to, 182

Anderson, D.D., Rev. James, officiates at Elizabeth Garrett's marriage ceremony, 186

Anderson, Dr. J. Ford, alluded to, 129, 199; a letter from Elizabeth Garrett Anderson quoted, 188, 189; quoted, on a speech of Elizabeth Garrett Anderson's, 261

Anderson, Mr. James George Skelton, meets Elizabeth Garrett, 129; and reforms of Shadwell Children's Hospital, *ib.*; letters from Elizabeth Garrett to, 131, 134, 137, 138, 140, 141, 143, 144, 150 *et seq.*, 160, 161, 168–74, 177 *et seq.*, 193–200, 202–4, 252–6; receives news of Elizabeth Garrett's Paris success, 132; the offices of, 142; visited in camp by Elizabeth Garrett, *ib.*; Emily Davies meets, 142, 143; Elizabeth Garrett criticizes the table talk of, 143; the parents of, 144, 145; education of, 145; joins firm of George Thomson & Co., 146; Elizabeth Garrett makes acquaintance of, *ib.*; and Elizabeth Garrett's School Board election Committee, 148, 149; a rebuking letter to Elizabeth Garrett from, 152; introduced to Aldeburgh, 162, 166; is engaged to Elizabeth Garrett, 163, 169; his father's enconiums of, 165; his conquest of Alde House, 166; Elizabeth Garrett proposes her rights in marriage to, 168, 169; Elizabeth Garrett to, on their future, 171, 172; his letter to Elizabeth Garrett, on their marriage, 175, 176; Newsom Garrett's cordiality towards, 178; a letter from Mrs. Garrett quoted, to, 180, 181; his gifts to Elizabeth Garrett, 181; Elizabeth Garrett to, on their independence, 182; unfriendly comments on

Index

the likely married status of, 184, 185; his characteristics and Elizabeth Garrett's compared, 185; letter to Elizabeth Garrett, on the sufficiency of their love, 185, 186; the Married Women's Property Act (1869) and, 186; his marriage to Elizabeth Garrett, *ib.*; first married years of, 188 *et seq.*; his affection for, and support of, his wife, 189; and Hitchin College, 189, 190; a letter on Hitchin College to, 190; the brief honeymoon of, 191; loyalty to his wife of, *ib.*; the children of, 192 & *n.*, 225; visits to Glasgow of, 192, 196, 197, 198, 202; his daughter Margaret dies, 201; as a guarantor for the London School of Medicine for Women, 225; removes to Aldeburgh, 239, 264; takes his wife and children to Australia, 245; a retrospective glance at the domestic life of, 264 *et seq.*; and Elizabeth Garrett Anderson's joy in a grandchild, 272; death of, *ib.*; a reminiscence of, as magistrate, *ib.*; Elizabeth Garrett Anderson succeeds as Mayor, 272, 273

Anderson, Louisa Garrett (after Doctor), alluded to, 192 *n.*, 194, 195, 196, 197, 198, 199, 202, 204, 227, 276; a letter to her mother quoted, 266, 267; and the War of 1914, 275

Anderson, Margaret Skelton, 192 *n.*, 194, 195; illness of, 198, 199; death of, 200, 201

Anderson, Mrs., 145

Anstie, Dr., 213, 216, 217, 218

Antwerp, Elizabeth Garrett sails for, 139; alluded to, 140

Apothecaries, The Society of, alluded to, 117, 207; Elizabeth Garrett obtains the L.S.A. diploma of, 118; alters its regulations, *ib.*; refuses to recognize the London School of Medicine for Women, 217

Apothecaries' Hall, The, Mr. Plaskitt alludes to, 85; the qualifying examination at, 87, 88; refuses application to compete for midwifery diploma, 94; rescinds its refusal, *ib.*; and Scottish University lectures, 97; Elizabeth Garrett and the examination of, 107; Elizabeth Garrett obtains the L.S.A. diploma of, 118; the licence to practice of, 130

Arlon, 139, 140

Armitage (artist), Mr., 161

Arnold (1795–1842), Thomas, alluded to, 118, 119

Atkins, M.D., Miss Louisa, 243

Atkins, Mrs., and New Hospital for Women, 245

Attorney General (*see* Kelly, Sir Fitzroy)

Australia, Elizabeth Garrett Anderson goes to, 245

Austria, Garibaldi and, 37

Bach Society, The, 83

Bacteriology, in 1860, 52

Barham (stockman), 35

Barnett (a maid), 182

Barnett, Rev. S. A. (after Canon), alluded to, 147, a biographical note of, *app.* 288

317

Index

Barry, Dr., 159

Bastian, F.R.S., Charlton, 147

Bayswater, letters from, 51, 55, 56, 59, 61, 62; Elizabeth Garrett at St. Agnes Villas in, 59

Beckar, Lydia, 146

Beesly, Professor, 143

Beilby, Miss, and a successful medical treatment of a Maharanee, 235

Beverley, Dr. Michael, 262

Bible, The, 36, 119

Bibliography, app. 311, 312

Bicycle, the, and women's dress reform, 24

Blackheath, Elizabeth Garrett at the Academy for Daughters of Gentlemen at, 32, 39

Blackwell, Dr. Elizabeth, meets Elizabeth Garrett, 42; Elizabeth Garrett attends lectures of, 42, 43; alluded to, 51, 206; a letter alluded to, 76; advises Elizabeth Garrett, *ib.*; and Elizabeth Garrett's admission as a student, 78; a letter from Elizabeth Garrett to, 93–6; and the Contagious Diseases Acts, 127; and the London School of Medicine for Women, 215; a biographical note of, *app.* 288

Blake, Miss L. B. Aldrich, 237, 239, 240

'Blue-stockings', 20

Blythe, Miss, 71

Bodichon, Mme Barbara L., alluded to, 23, 42; Emily Davies meets, 41; the education of, *ib.*; Elizabeth Blackwell and Elizabeth Garrett at house of, 42; the bureau for women of, 91; and

the franchise, 121; and a Westminster election, *ib.*; and the Women's Petition (1866), 122; supports Elizabeth Garrett's candidature for the School Board, 147; a biographical note of, *app.* 289

Bolton, C.B.E., M.D., Miss Elizabeth, 11

Bombay, Drs. Pechy and Hitchcock work in, 236; Mr. Cama's Hospital for Women at, *ib.*; the University of, *ib.*

Bonn University, 145

Bouillon, 140

Box Hill (Dorking), 175

Bow, 178

Bright, Rt. Hon. John, 222

British Medical Association, The, Elizabeth Garrett and membership of, 251; women and membership of, *ib.*; criticism of women's membership of, 251–255; Elizabeth Garrett Anderson's election to, 256; Mrs. Hoggan and, *ib.*; a plebiscite on women's admission to, *ib.*; Elizabeth Garrett Anderson on women and, 257–61; the motion against women members of, 261; the clause against women expunged, 262; Elizabeth Garrett Anderson elected President of the East Anglian branch of, *ib.*

British Medical Journal, The, quoted, 55; and Elizabeth Garrett's Paris success, 132, 133; and women's membership of the B.M.A., 253; Elizabeth Garrett Anderson on women and the B.M.A. quoted, 257–61; on Elizabeth Garrett

Index

Anderson's presidential speech to B.M.A., 262, 263

British Medical Register, The, foreign degrees not recognized by, 130; women on (1878), *app.* 285

Broadbent, Sir William, 198, 199, 200, 241

Brooks, Miss L. M., 240

Browning, Miss, her school at Blackheath, 32, 33

Browning, Robert, and the School Board election campaign, 148; alluded to, 158

Brudenell Terrace (Aldeburgh), Newson Garrett builds, 30

Brussels, Elizabeth Garrett travels to, 138

Buchanan, Dr., 216, 233

Burt, Miss, 11

Buss, Miss, supports Elizabeth Garrett's candidature for School Board, 147

Butler, Miss Fanny, 218

Butler, Mrs. Josephine, and the Contagious Diseases Acts, 127, 128; a biographical note of (*Life* cited), *app.* 289

Caldesi (photographer), 161, 162

Cama, Mr., his Hospital at Bombay for women, 236

Cambridge, University of, 32, 77, 96; the Classical Tripos at, 232

Cameron, Dr., 222

Campbell, Professor Lewis, and Elizabeth Garrett's engagement, 164

Canton, Dr., a letter of Elizabeth Garrett's to, 107, 108

Cassandra (Florence Nightingale), alluded to, 10, 22

Chambers, Dr. King, 221

Chambers's Encyclopaedia, cited, *app.* 294, *app.* 306

Chanonry (Old Aberdeen), 144; Rev. Alexander Anderson's Gymnasium at, 145

Cheadle, Dr., 216

Children, husband's and wife's rights over (1836), 19; the Equal Guardianship of Infants Act, *ib.*; baptismal immersion of in Scotland, 144; of Rev. Alexander Anderson, 145; of Elizabeth Garrett Anderson, 192 *& n.*, 245, 266; Mrs. Anderson's nurse and, 192, 194, 195, 196, 197–200; death of Margaret Skelton Anderson, 200; Elizabeth Garrett Anderson's treatment of her own, 269; the Garrett family, *app.* 279

Christ Church (Marylebone), 70, 73, 74

Christie, Mr., 148, 153

Christison, Sir Robert, his hostility to women students, 208; a libel action by, 208, 209; opposes women's membership of the B.M.A., 252, 253

Church Hill (Aldeburgh), the Garrett's house on, 27

City of London School, The, 32

Clapham, 223

Clark, Sir Andrew, supports Elizabeth Garrett's candidature for the School Board, 147; alluded to, 170, 237

Coach travel, 23, 24

Index

Cobbe, Miss Frances Power, 143; a biographical note of, *app.* 290

Cobden, Richard, 93

Cock, Dr. Julia, appointed sub-Dean of London School of Medicine for Women, 237; succeeds Elizabeth Garrett Anderson as Dean, 239; alluded to, 240, 248, 268; death of, 240

Col (a collie dog), 204

Colin (Elizabeth Garrett Anderson's grandson), 276

Collards, Messrs., Elizabeth Garrett addresses employees of, 151, 152

College of Physicians, The Royal, 77; refuses to recognize the London School of Medicine for Women, 217; of Ireland, 222

College of Surgeons, The Royal, refuses Elizabeth Garrett's application to compete for diploma, 94; refuses to recognize the London School of Medicine for Women, 217; a tumour offered to the Museum of, 245

Comte, 124

Contagious Diseases Acts, The, 127; Elizabeth Garrett and, 127, 128; the repeal of, 128

Cornhill (London), 177, 179, 180

Cotton, Alderman, 159

Court, The Royal, Elizabeth Garrett Anderson presented at, 269

Courtney, Leonard Henry, Baron, supports Elizabeth Garrett's candidature for the School Board, 147; a biographical note of, *app.* 290

Cowell, Mrs. Herbert, alluded to, 34, 38, 166, 193; Elizabeth Garrett announces her intention to be a doctor to, 43; Elizabeth Garrett quoted, to, 125; takes Elizabeth Garrett's place on the London School Board, 191

Cowell, Philip, 265

Crabbe, George, 27; a biographical note of, *app.* 291

Crimean War, The, 37, 46

Critchett, Mr., 216, 241

Crowe, Miss Annie, Elizabeth Garrett visits, 39

Crowe, Miss Jane, Elizabeth Garrett visits, 39; alluded to, 74, 80, 143; and the women's movement, 91

Daily News, The, 160

Davies, Rev. J. Llewelyn, alluded to, 40, 74; introduces Elizabeth Garrett to Mrs. Russell Gurney, 51; supports the women's movement, 73; his friendship with Elizabeth Garrett, *ib.*; supports Elizabeth Garrett's candidature for School Board, 147; and Elizabeth Garrett's engagement, 164; and St. Mary's Dispensary, 241, 242; accepts living of Kirby Lonsdale, 265; death of, 267; a biographical note of, *app.* 291, 292

Davies, Mrs. Llewelyn, entertains Elizabeth Garrett, 75; removes to Kirby Lonsdale, 265; death of, 266; alluded to, 268

Davies, Margaret Llewelyn, alluded to, 9, 265; Elizabeth Garrett Anderson quoted, to, 266; a letter in tribute to her father quoted, 267

Index

Davies, Miss Sarah Emily, her letters to Elizabeth Garrett alluded to, 9; *Emily Davies and Girton College (vide)*, 9; and women's repression, 23; Elizabeth Garrett's first meeting with, 39; her influence upon Elizabeth Garrett, *ib.*; her attitude to the position of women, 40; quoted, on women's aimlessness, *ib.*; the neglected education of, 40; women in the medical profession and, 41; meets Mme Bodichon and her sisters, *ib.*; her second meeting with Elizabeth Garrett, *ib.*; personal impression of, 42; Elizabeth Garrett impressed by, 43; her correspondence with Elizabeth Garrett, 43–7, 51, 52, 58, 59, 61, 62, 68, 69, 72, 73, 86, 87, 88, 109–13, 118, 119, 147, 163; helps Elizabeth Garrett with criticism, 44, 45; letters alluded to, 47; her visits to Alde House, 47, 48; and Girton, 48; characteristics of, *ib.*; a reminiscence of Elizabeth Garrett and, 48, 49; advises Elizabeth Garrett meeting Mrs. Russell Gurney, 51; advised by Elizabeth Garrett of her father's sanction, 56; her advice on being 'lady-like', 63; advises Elizabeth Garrett against a tutor, 70, 71; Elizabeth Garrett's letter on the Medical School's opposition, to, 82, 83; Elizabeth Garrett announces the Medical School's decision, to, 84; and Mme Bodichon, 91; a letter to Lady Stephen quoted, 91, 92; and the new Charter of the University of London, 93; joins and assists Elizabeth Garrett at St. Andrews, 106; Elizabeth Garrett quoted, to, 108; on Elizabeth Garrett's neglect of advice, 114, 115, 116; and Hitchin College, 117, 189; her interest in the women's movement, 117; and the franchise, 121, 122, 124; visits the Wimbledon camp, 142; the School Board candidature of, 146, 149; her friendly help to Elizabeth Garrett alluded to, 150, 268; opposes Elizabeth Garrett for Chairman of the School Board, 157; alluded to, 158, 159, 170, 267, *app.* 284; congratulates Elizabeth Garrett on her engagement, 163, 164; fewer meetings between Elizabeth Garrett Anderson and, 190; a biographical note of, *app.* 292, 293

Day (St. Andrews), Dr., offers to help Elizabeth Garrett, 89; reluctance of, 90; advises Elizabeth Garrett, 98, 99; the secretary of, 98, 99; alluded to, 100, 103, 105, 106; enlists Dr. Tulloch's support, 102; Elizabeth Garrett works privately under, 106

de la Cherois, Mrs., 245, 248

De Morgan (hospital treasurer), Mr., 56, 65, 66, 70; the opposition of, 77, 78

Denham, Q. C., The Hon. John, 123

Dewar (nurse), Mrs., 194

Dictionary of National Biography, The, cited, *app.* 287–310

Index

Disraeli, Benjamin, 122

Disruption of Scottish Church (1843), The, 144, 145

Dissecting, 75, 76; Elizabeth Garrett and, 77; Elizabeth Garrett's need for experience in, 107

Don (Alan Garrett Anderson's dog), 267, 271

Dove, Miss Frances, 266, 267

Dover, the Lord Warden hotel at, 205

Dowler, Rev. Mr., alluded to, 28, 91; Elizabeth Garrett comments on sermons of, 45

Drewry, Miss Ellen, 65, 68, 72, 89 90

Dreyfus case, The, 265

Dufferin, The Countess of, starts the Female Medical Supply (India) Association, 236

Duncan, M., 253, 255

Dunnell, Louisa (*see* Garrett, Mrs. Newson)

East London Hospital for Children (Shadwell), The, (after The Princess Elizabeth of York Hospital for Children); Elizabeth Garrett and a vacancy on medical staff of, 128, 129; Elizabeth Garrett appointed to medical staff of, 129, *app*. 283; Elizabeth Garrett, Mr. Anderson, and reforms of, 129, 137, 146; a letter of Elizabeth Garrett's on, 138, 140; efforts to improve, 142; Mr. Anderson on the Board of, 149; the out-patient department of, 177, 179; alluded to, 178, 179; Elizabeth Garrett Anderson resigns from medical staff of, 191,

192; the Minute Book quoted, *app*. 283

Edgeworth (governess), Miss, and the Garretts, 30, 31; described, 31; the school books of, *ib*.; and the Garrett children, *ib*.; alluded to, 33

Edinburgh, alluded to, 98, 223; Elizabeth Garrett works under Professor Simpson and Dr. Keiller at, 107; School Boards and, 146; Elizabeth Garrett Anderson's letters from, on women and the British Medical Association, 252–6

Edinburgh, University of, refuses Elizabeth Garrett as a student, 107; women studying medicine at, 133; students congratulate Elizabeth Garrett, 134; Sophia Jex-Blake and matriculation at, 206; Elizabeth Garrett and women students at, 207; hostility of Faculty of Medicine to women students, 208, 210; champions of women students at, 209; Sophia Jex-Blake withdraws from, 210; women who matriculated at (1869), *app*. 285

Education, of women, 20, 22; Newson Garrett and, 29; Emily Davies, on women's, 40; Rev. Alexander Anderson's school at Chanonry, 145; Mr. Forster's Education Act, 146; School Boards and elementary, 146; foreign, 210

Eliot, George, 124; *The Spanish Gipsy*, poem alluded to, 164, 173

Index

Elizabeth Garrett Anderson Hospital, The (previously New Hospital for Women), alluded to, 250

Ellaby, Dr. Charlotte, 248

Ellis, Mrs., quoted, on married women, 21, 22

Emily Davies and Girton College, 9, 91, 92, 121, 149, *app.* 287, 289, 293

Equal Guardianship of Infants Act (1839), The, 19

Erichsen, on operations, 54, 55

Eton, Alan Garrett Anderson at, 267

Eyre Arms, The, Elizabeth Garrett's School Board election meeting at, 152

Faithfull, Miss Emily, 91; a biographical note of, *app.* 293

Family Chronicle, The, quoted, 121

Fawcett, Professor Henry, alluded to, 135, 147, 167, 187, 225, 265; a biographical note of, *app.* 293, 294

Fawcett, Mrs. Millicent, alluded to, 34, 37, 38, 166, 265; at a Suffrage meeting, 135; an experience of, *ib.*; a letter of Elizabeth Garrett's to, 167, 168, 201; and Elizabeth Garrett's wedding, 187; goes to Rome, 193, 195; a letter from, quoted, 267; and Women's Suffrage, 273; a biographical note of, *app.* 295; *What I Remember*, cited, *app.* 295

Fawcett, Philippa, 265

Firth of Forth, The, 98

Fleury, Miss, the Irish University success of, 232

Florence, a letter from, 194

Flower, F.R.S., V. H., supports Elizabeth Garrett's candidature for School Board, 147

Forbes, Principal, 103

Forster, Mr. W. E., the Education Act of, 146

Fowler, Dr., 80

France, Anatole, *Thaïs* disliked by Elizabeth Garrett Anderson, 270

Franchise, The Parliamentary, alluded to, 18; in 1865, 120; John Stuart Mill's views on women and, 120, 121; Elizabeth Garrett's interest in, 134; the School Board Election and, 156

Franco-German War, The, outbreak of, 137; Elizabeth Garrett's sympathy with France in, 138; the German victories in, *ib.*; Elizabeth Garrett goes to the war zone, 139; Elizabeth Garrett's experiences in, 140, 141; Elizabeth Garrett and a helpful Prussian officer, 140–2; the German advance and siege of Paris, 142; Elizabeth Garrett and two American fugitives from, 142

Freeman, Mrs. Sarah, 51

Freeman, Mr. William, 58

Galton, Dr. J. H., champions women's cause against the B.M.A., 262

Garibaldi, General, 195

Garrett, Agnes, 166

Garrett, Alice (*see* Cowell, Mrs. Herbert)

Garrett, Edmund, 32, 37, 38, 154

Garrett, George, 37

Index

Garrett, Josephine, 138, 139, 140, 165, 166

Garrett, Louisa Maria (*see* Smith, Mrs. J.W.)

Garrett, Millicent (*see* Fawcett, Mrs. Millicent)

Garrett, Mrs. Newson (*née* Louisa Dunnell), Elizabeth Garrett born to, 25, 26; marriage of, 26; the children of, 26, *app.* 279; at Aldeburgh, 26; the Aldeburgh home of, 27; her petty cash book quoted, 27, 28; her husband's need of, 28; the correspondence of, *ib.*; the piety of, 29; the first cheque book of, *ib.*; a governess appointed by, 30-2; breakfast prayers of, 36; is opposed to Elizabeth's choice of the medical profession, 47, 50; depression of, 61; alluded to, 71, 100; recalls her daughter Louisa, 126; meets Mr. Anderson, 162, 166; a letter to Mr. Anderson quoted, 180, 181; letters from Elizabeth Garrett Anderson quoted, 247; entertains the British Medical Association doctors, 263; Elizabeth Garrett Anderson's correspondence with, 264; the family of, *app.* 279

Garrett, Mr. Newson, the forebears of, 25; birth of, 26; children of, 26, *app.* 279; his home at Aldeburgh, 26, 27; his life at Aldeburgh, 28; and his wife, 28, 29; education of, 29; activities of, 29, 30; as Justice of the Peace, 30; his death alluded to, *ib.*; and his children's education, 32; his progress at Aldeburgh, 35;

builds Alde House, *ib.*; reminiscences of, 35, 36; political keenness of, 37; political coolness between Richard Garrett and, 37; assists Elizabeth Garrett with pocket money, 39; and Elizabeth Garrett's choice of the medical profession, 43, 44; reluctantly supports Elizabeth's medical aspirations, 50; interviews Harley Street consultants, *ib.*; a letter to Elizabeth Garrett quoted, 56; Elizabeth Garrett alludes to, 60, 72; Elizabeth Garrett asks advice of, 71; and his daughter's plans, 87, 90; petitions University of London in behalf of women, 93; consults Justice Hannen, 97; his kind letters to Elizabeth Garrett, 101; threatens legal action against Society of Apothecaries, 117; meets Mr. Anderson, 162; and Elizabeth Garrett's engagement, 165, 166; letters from Elizabeth Garrett to, 233, 236, 238, 249; death of, 263; as Mayor of Aldeburgh, *ib.*; the family of, *app.* 279, 280

Garrett (1675), Richard, 25

Garrett, Richard, 25, 26, 33; a political coolness with Newson Garrett, 37

Garrett, Mrs. Richard, Elizabeth Garrett's letters to, 57, 58; advises Elizabeth Garrett against medical training, 58

Garrett, Samuel, 32, 138

Gateshead, Elizabeth Garrett visits school-friends at, 39, 41; Elizabeth Garrett and Emily Davies at, 39; alluded to, 43

Index

Geddes, Mrs. Auckland, 146

General Medical Council, The, the Government's application to regarding the profession, 220

Germany, Elizabeth Garrett Anderson in, 265 (see also Franco-German War)

Germany, Universities of, 130, 145

Girton College, Emily Davies and, 48; the first mistress of, 189

Gladstone, Mr. W. E., 93, 264, 270

Glasgow, 192, 196, 197, 198

Glasgow, University of, 97, 233

Glenham, 25

Grafton Hall (Tottenham Court Road), 151

Granville, Lord, 96, 191, 233; an interview with Elizabeth Garrett Anderson, 226, 227; a biographical note of, app. 301

Graves (Dublin), Dr., alluded to, 132

Great Exhibition in Hyde Park (1851), The, Elizabeth Garrett views, 33, 34

Greenwich, 146, 149, app. 284

Gregory, Dr. Hazel Chodak, 192

Grote, George, a biographical note of, app. 295

Grote, Mrs. Harriet, her assistance to Elizabeth Garrett, 95; alluded to, 112; at a Women's Suffrage meeting, 135; the conversion to enfranchisement of, ib.; an impression of, 136; a biographical note of, app. 296, 297

Grundy, Mrs., 162

Guildhall (London), The, 156, 179, 182

Gurney, Mrs. Russell, Elizabeth Garrett meets, 51; alluded to, 55, 56, 75, 93, 130, 249, 268; on feminine arts, 77, 79; and the Medical Schools' rejection of Elizabeth Garrett, 84; a letter to Elizabeth Garrett quoted, 84, 85; a consoling letter to Elizabeth Garrett, 106; an encouraging letter to Elizabeth Garrett from, 132; in praise of Elizabeth Garrett's influence, 136; and the School Board election result, 156, 158; a letter alluded to, 169; death of, 248; her legacy to New Hospital for Women, ib.

Gurney, Rt. Hon. Russell, alluded to, 55, 84, 249; his Bill for women's right to medical examinations, 222; a letter quoted, ib.; the Enabling Act of, 245; a biographical note of, app. 297

Hall, Lady, 250

Hall (Deputy Mayor of Aldeburgh), Mr., 274

Hammond, J. L., and Barbara, Life of Lord Shaftesbury, cited, app. 306; Life of Stansfeld, app. 310

Hampstead, 150, 156, 173

Hannay, Professor R. K., 10

Hannen, Mr. Justice, his letters on University charters and women, 97; supports Elizabeth Garrett's candidature for School Board, 147; a biographical note of, app. 297, 298

Hanover Square Rooms, The, women's suffrage meeting in, 135

Harley Street, Newson Garrett interviews doctors of, 50; Queen's College for Women in, 68

Index

Hart, Dr. Ernest, 133, 252

Haweis, Rev. H. R., supports Elizabeth Garrett's candidature for School Board, 147; a biographical note of, *app.* 298

Hawes, Mr. William, 52, 55, 64

Heckford, Dr., 110, 111, 112, 128, *app.* 283

Heddle (St. Andrews), Dr., 98, 100, 103

Heisch, Mr., 82, 86

Henrietta Street, No. 30, lease purchased by Miss Jex-Blake, 217

Herford, Miss Laura, her portrait of Elizabeth Garrett alluded to, 43

Hern, Mr. William, 10

Hesperus, S.S., 193

Higher Local University Examinations, The, 117

Hill (Editor), Mr., 124

Hill, Mr. Hay, 148, 154

Hill, Miss Miranda, 89

Hill, Miss Octavia, supports Elizabeth Garrett's candidature for School Board, 147; a biographical note of, *app.* 298

Hitchcock, Dr. 236

Hitchin College, Emily Davies and, 117, 189

Hoggan, Mrs. 242, 244, 253, 255, 256

Home Quartet Society, The, Elizabeth Garrett Anderson a founder of, 203

Hope Scholarship for Chemistry (Edinburgh), The, 208

Hopgood, Mr. and Mrs. James, 223, 225

House of Commons, The, the Women's petition (1866) presented in, 122; and the Contagious Diseases Acts, 127; and Women's Suffrage, 274

Hughes, Thomas, 75; a biographical note of, *app.* 299

Humanitarian movement, the, 18

Hungry Forties, The, 37

Huxley, Professor T. H., Elizabeth Garrett attends lectures of, 89; supports women's enfranchisement, 122; alluded to, 147; and the School Board election, 154, 155; and the School Board chairmanship, 159; becomes a Governor of the London School of Medicine for Women, 219; a biographical note of, *app.* 299, 300

Hyde Park, the 1851 Exhibition in, 33, 34

Hygienic Congress (1891), The, 128

India, medical women in, 234-6

Indian Female Evangelist, The, 234

Indian Mutiny, The, 37

Ipswich, 32

Ireland, the potato famine in, 37

Italy, Garibaldi and, 37; Elizabeth Garrett Anderson in, 194-6, 205

Jackson, Mrs., Elizabeth Garrett's letter to, on School Board election committee, 148

Jackson, Dr. Hughlings, 241

Jenner, Miss, 226

Jenner, Sir William, 226

Jews, the, 29

Jex-Blake, F.R.C.P., Dr. Arthur, 11

Index

Jex-Blake, Sophia, alluded to, 11, 89, 91, 133, 252; the circle of, 90; letter to Elizabeth Garrett quoted, 126; congratulates Elizabeth Garrett on the M.D. success, 133; and the London School of Medicine for Women, 205, 213 et seq.; at Queen's College, 206; Elizabeth Garrett and, 207, 210; a libel action against, 208, 209; her action against the Edinburgh Senatus, 209; withdraws from Edinburgh, 210; Life of, 210, 212, 215, 223, 224, 228, app. 300, 301, app. 309, 310; replies to Elizabeth Garrett Anderson's Times letter, 212, 213; founds the London School of Medicine for Women, 213–15; letter to Elizabeth Garrett Anderson on London School of Medicine for Women, 214, 215; the ruling spirit of the London School of Medicine for Women, 216, 217; purchases lease of 30 Henrietta Street, 217; a member of deputation from London School of Medicine to Government, 221; a letter from Mr. Russell Gurney quoted, 222; introduces Sir James Stansfeld to London School of Medicine, 223, Sir James Stansfeld and the Royal Free Hospital's assent, 224; resigns as Trustee of London School of Medicine for Women, 227, 228; Elizabeth Garrett Anderson and the resignation of, 229; a biographical note of (Life cited), app. 300

Keiller (Edinburgh), Dr., 107, 255
Kelly, Sir Fitzroy, 37; and the London University charter, 95; the unfavourable opinion of, 104, 105
Kirby Lonsdale, Rev. Llewelyn Davies goes to, 265, 266

'La Migraine', Elizabeth Garrett's Paris thesis on, 132
Lambert (coachman), 35, 166
Lancet, The, an unfriendly article alluded to, 85; opposes women's entry into the medical schools, 94; quoted, app. 282
Langham Place, Mme Bodichon's office in, 91, 121
Law (editor), Mr. William, 209
Law Society, The, 32
Lawrence, Lord, 157
Lawrence, Mr. and Mrs. Pethick, 274
Leiston, Garrett & Sons' works at, 25, 34
Leith Hill, 175
Life of Sophia Jex-Blake, The, 210, 212, 215, 223, 224, 228
Lime Street Square, Mr. Anderson's offices in, 142
Lind, Miss Jenny, 158; a biographical note of, app. 301, 302
Lister, Joseph, alluded to, 11; and Pasteur's germ theory, 53; quoted, to Pasteur, 53, 54; St. Clair Thomson's tribute to, 54
Lockyer, Sir Joseph Norman, supports Elizabeth Garrett's candidature for School Board, 147; a biographical note of, app. 302

Index

Loftie, Rev. W. J., supports Elizabeth Garrett's candidature for School Board, 147; a biographical note of, *app.* 302

London, the Garretts live in, 26; alluded to, 32, 47, 210, 223, 265; Louisa Garrett in, 36; Elizabeth Garrett meets Dr. E. Blackwell in, 42; letters from, 196–200, 202–4; Newson and Elizabeth Garrett consult doctors in, 50; Elizabeth Garrett comes to, 59, 107; Professor Huxley lectures in, 89; Elizabeth Garrett returns to, 90; letters from Elizabeth Garrett in, 109–13

London, University of, Elizabeth Garrett's plan to matriculate at, 87, 89; the new Charter of, 93, 95, 96, 191; Elizabeth Garrett and, 93; Elizabeth Garrett prepares to matriculate at, 93; the Vice-Chancellor of, 95; Miss Edith Shove and, 226, 232; the new charter and admission of women to, 226; the London School of Medicine for Women, a college of, 230; first women M.D.s of, 233; and the students of New Hospital for Women, 239

London Hospital, The, Elizabeth Garrett visits wards of, 110, 111; opposition to Elizabeth Garrett at, 112; Elizabeth Garrett expelled from, 113; Mr. Heckford's connection with, 129; refuses recognition of the London School of Medicine for Women, 218, 219

London School of Medicine for Women, The, Miss Jex-Blake and, 205, 213 *et seq.*, 227, 228; first teaching staff of, 213; Elizabeth Garrett Anderson and, 214, 215, 216; Elizabeth Garrett Anderson and the Council of, 215; the first offices of, 216; the provisional Council of, *ib.*; the first students of, 218, 225; refusals of recognition of, *ib.*; the London and Royal Free Hospitals refuse recognition of, 218, 219; the body of Governors of, 219, Elizabeth Garrett Anderson; elected a lecturer in medicine at, 219; the Executive Council and decreasing students of, 220; Elizabeth Garrett Anderson a member of a deputation to Government from, 221; listed as a recognized medical school, 223; Royal Free Hospital assents to clinical teaching of students of, 224; subscriptions to, and appeal for funds by, 225; the first bequest to, 226; Mrs. Thorne appointed Hon. Sec. to, 227; Miss Jex-Blake resigns as trustee of, 228; and Miss Jex-Blake's resignation, 229; Elizabeth Garrett Anderson succeeds as Dean of, 229–33; the register of, 231; missionaries of, 234; progress of, 236; Miss Julia Cock and, 237; increase of students at, 237, 238; the rebuilding of, 238, 240; affiliated to London University, 239; Elizabeth Garrett Anderson resigns office of Dean of, *ib.*; Treasury grants to, 240; alluded to, 265; students attending (1887–1917), *app.* 286

Index

London Scottish Regiment, The, 142

Lorimer (Aaa), Nurse Helen, 192, 193, 196, 197, 200, 204

Louise, Princess, 130

Lucknow, 235

Lyons, Lord, 130

McBean, Mr., 99, 101

Macdonald (St. Andrews), Professor William, 103

Madras, 236

Manchester, 146

Manchester Square, 70, 71; Elizabeth Garrett removes to, 72; letters from, 73, 76–82, 93–6; Mrs. Smith's (Louisa Garrett) house in, 90, 107, 113

Mansion House, The, Elizabeth Garrett's School Board election meeting at, 153; New Hospital for Women appeal meeting at, 246

Marlborough House, Mrs. Scharlieb received at, 236

Marriage, of Elizabeth Garrett and Mr. J. G. S. Anderson, 186, 187; the Anderson's first years of, 188 et seq.; Elizabeth Garrett Anderson's happiness in, 188, 189; Elizabeth Garrett Anderson's busy life after, 191

Married Women's Property Acts, The, 19; Elizabeth Garrett and, 186

Marshall, Mrs., 245, 247, 248, 252, 255, 262

Marshall, Dr. William, 254

Mary, H.M. Queen, 240

Marylebone, Working Men's Association in, 147; Elizabeth Garrett canvasses, 150; Elizabeth

Garrett married in, 186; alluded to, app. 284

Masson, Mrs., 223

Masson, Professor David, supports Elizabeth Garrett's candidature for School Board, 147; champions women medical students, 209, 223; a biographical note of, app. 303

Maud, Princess, 247

Maurice, The Rev. F.D., his sympathy with the women's movement, 68, 69; colleges founded by, 69; and Elizabeth Garrett, 69, 206; alluded to, 73, 75, 110; Elizabeth Garrett and the sermons of, 91; a biographical note (Life cited), app. 303

Medical Acts, The, of 1858, 42, 211, 213; of 1876, 222

M.D. degree, the, Elizabeth Garrett and, 95, 96; of Paris, 129 et seq., app. 282

Medical Practice, Elizabeth Garrett begins, 120; Elizabeth Garrett's increase in, 128; Elizabeth Garrett's consultants in, 136; growth of, after Elizabeth Garrett's marriage, 191, women in, 206

Medical Profession, The, Emily Davies's plans for women in, 41; Elizabeth Garrett's choice of, and training for, 50 et seq.; the General Medical Council report to Government on women and, 220

Medical Register, The, Dr. Elizabeth Blackwell placed on, 42; women and, 210; alluded to, 259; women and (1878), app. 285

Medical School, The Middlesex Hospital, alluded to, 64; opposition to Elizabeth Garrett at, 77; students' petition for dismissal of Elizabeth Garrett, 80–4; Elizabeth Garrett appeals to students of, 81, 82; reply to Elizabeth Garrett by students of, 83; Elizabeth Garrett refused admittance into, 84, 86; decides against Elizabeth Garrett, 84; Elizabeth Garrett leaves, 86; its hostile opposition to Elizabeth Garrett, 92

Medical Schools, their hostile opposition to Elizabeth Garrett, 92, 94; theWestminster Hospital, 94; the London Hospitals, *ib.*; the Grosvenor Street, *ib.*; the London School for women, 205, 206 *et seq.*

Medical Training, in a surgical ward, 52, 53; Elizabeth Garrett begins, 55; Elizabeth Garrett at Middlesex Hospital, 59, 60, 62, 65; Elizabeth Garrett aspires to studentship, 63, 65, 67, 69, 70; Elizabeth Garrett and night nursing, 66, 68, 71; Elizabeth Garrett receives first lessons in, 72; Elizabeth Garrett and dissecting, 75, 76, 77, 79; lectures and Elizabeth Garrett, 76, 77, 78, 79; Elizabeth Garrett and examinations in, 80; students' petition for dismissal of Elizabeth Garrett, 80, 81, 82, 83, 84; a break in Elizabeth Garrett's, 86; refused to Elizabeth Garrett, 93, 94; refused to compete for midwifery diploma, 94; efforts for

women in, 94, 95, 96; Justice Hannen on universities and women for, 97; Elizabeth Garrett rebuffed by St. Andrews, 105, 107; the London Hospital and Elizabeth Garrett, 110–13; Elizabeth Garrett's efforts to continue, 92, 93; Sophia Jex-Blake applies for, 206; the London School of Medicine for Women, 206 *et seq.*; Edinburgh refuses women for, 208

'*Medicine as a Profession for Ladies*', Dr. Elizabeth Blackwell lectures on, 42

Meredith, Dr., 244

Metz, 141

Middlesex Hospital, the surgery ward at, 52, 53; Elizabeth Garrett goes to, 55; Elizabeth Garrett trains as nurse at, 58; Elizabeth Garrett enters, 59; Elizabeth Garrett's first duties at, 60; discreet manner of Elizabeth Garrett at, 62; Elizabeth Garrett, on the help of Mr. Willis at, 62; the Medical College of (*vide*); the Governing Board of, 64; Elizabeth Garrett at, 64, 65, 128; letters from, 64, 65, 66, 67, 68, 69, 75; Elizabeth Garrett and studentship at, 65; Elizabeth Garrett on night duty at, 66; Elizabeth Garrett on fees of, 66; Elizabeth Garrett as apothecary's pupil at, 66, 67; the resident medical officer at, 67; Elizabeth Garrett dissects at, 75; diagnosis at, 75, 76; Elizabeth Garrett and the opposition of the Medical School of, 77, 92, 112; Elizabeth

Index

Garrett's progress at, 79; Elizabeth Garrett leaves, 86; hostile opposition to Elizabeth Garrett at, 92; Elizabeth Garrett's friends at, 113; Elizabeth Garrett visits wards at, 113, 114; her visiting the wards ends, 114; Elizabeth Garrett's consultants usually of, 136; the staff of (1860), *app.* 280, 281

Mill, John Stuart, political views of, 120; and the parliamentary franchise, 121; the enfranchisement petition of, 121, 135; visited by Lord and Lady Amberley, 124

Missionaries, opposition to supplying medical knowledge to, 234

Möhl, Lady, 158

Möhl, Professor, 158; a biographical note of, *app.* 304

Moncrieff, Lord Advocate James, and women and the University charter, 105 & *n.*

Morgan, M.D., Miss (*see* Hoggan, Mrs.)

Morpeth, 186

Murchison, Dr., the incivility of, 80; alluded to, 177

Murray, Dr. Flora, 275

Murray, Dr. John, 128, 129

Napoleon Bonaparte, 27, 127

Napoleon III, The Emperor, 131

National Union of Women's Suffrage Societies, The, 134, 135, 273, 274

Nelaton, alluded to, 55

New Hospital for Women, The, started as St. Mary's Dispensary by Elizabeth Garrett, 120; Elizabeth Garrett's work at the Dispensary, 128; the dispensary of, 170; the growth of, 231; Elizabeth Garrett Anderson's appeals for, 232; the Prince and Princess of Wales's visit to, 238; the Earl of Shaftesbury and, 242; described, 242, 243; Elizabeth Garrett Anderson's surgical work at, 243; 'No men or no hospital', 244; ovariotomy operation performed by a woman at, *ib.*; increasing medical staff of, 245; visiting physicians at, *ib.*; Elizabeth Garrett Anderson on a successful operation at, 245, 246; a new site found for, 246; a public appeal for building, *ib.*; Florence Nightingale and, *ib.*; Princess of Wales lays the foundation stone of new buildings, 247; drawing-room meetings in behalf of, *ib.*; result of appeals for, *ib.*; the in- and out-patients' staff of, 248; the accommodation of the new building, *ib.*; Elizabeth Garrett Anderson resigns from visiting staff of, *ib.*; Mrs. Scharlieb, Miss Cock and, *ib.*; Mrs. Russell Gurney's legacy to, 248, 249; Elizabeth Garrett Anderson resigns Chairmanship of Committee of, 249; Mr. A. G. Pollock and, 249, 250; Alan Anderson and, 250; its name changed, *ib.*; the present accommodation of, *ib.*; alluded to, 265

Newman, Sir George, 240

Nightingale, Florence, *Cassandra* alluded to, 10; quoted, on women and marriage, 19; her

Index

school of nursing founded, 20; quoted, on women's repression, 22; early life of, *ib.*; alluded to, 246

Nightingale School of Nursing, The, 20

Norton, Dr. A. T., alluded to, 213, 216, 221, 241; as Dean of the London School of Medicine for Women, 218, 219; resigns as Dean, 228; Elizabeth Garrett Anderson succeeds as Dean of London School of Medicine, 229; quoted, 233

Norton, Mrs. Caroline, the case of, 18, 19, 23; a biographical note of, *app.* 304

Nottingham, the British Medical Association and women's membership, at, 262

Nunn, Dr. T. W., cordiality of, 59; his friendliness to Elizabeth Garrett, 60, 62, 78; alluded to, 64, 75, 79; Elizabeth Garrett's confidence in, 65; accepts Elizabeth Garrett as a private pupil, 69, 70; and Elizabeth Garrett's wish to dissect, 76; recommends chemistry lectures, *ib.*; withdraws consent to Elizabeth Garrett about dissecting, 79; and the Medical Schools' rejection of Elizabeth Garrett, 84

Nunn, Mrs., 69, 70

Nursing, the Nightingale School of (1860), 20; Elizabeth Garrett and, 50, 73; Elizabeth Garrett at London Hospital, 110

Oakes, Mrs. George, her bequest to London School of Medicine for Women, 228

Operations, mortality of (1860), 52, 53

Otté, Miss, 98, 99, 105

Oxford, University of, 96

Paddington, 156; the British Medical Association's branch at, 251, 252

Paget, Bt., Sir James, on public life and marriage of Elizabeth Garrett, 184

Pall Mall Gazette, The, 133, 134

Pankhurst, Miss Christabel, 274

Pankhurst, Mrs., alluded to, 273; and Votes for Women, 274

Paris, surgery during the siege of, 55; Elizabeth Garrett and the M.D. degree of, 129 *et seq., app.* 282; the British Ambassador in, 130; Elizabeth Garrett's visits to, 131; letter to Mr. Anderson from, *ib.*; the siege of, 142; alluded to, 210

Paris, University of, opens the M.D. degree to women, 130; Elizabeth Garrett sits for examination at, *ib.*; Elizabeth Garrett takes the M.D. degree of, 132, 133

Parliament, J. S. Mill, and a women's petition to, 121

Pasteur, Joseph Lister and, 53, 54; the *Life* of quoted, 53, 54

Pechy, Edith, alluded to, 208, 215, 216; a tribute to, 222; her work in Bombay, 236

Pemberton, Mr., his opposition to women members of the British Medical Association, 252, 253, 254

Pennington, Mr. Frederick, 225

Index

Penton, K.B.E., Sir Edward, 10
Persia, The Shah of, 264
Perugia, a letter from, 194
Peters (the Andersons' nurse), Annie, 144, 145; and Elizabeth Garrett's 'notoriety', 165
Philpot Street (London), Elizabeth Garrett's lodgings in, and letters from, 110–13
Pio Nono, His Holiness Pope, 195
Plaskitt, Dr., Elizabeth Garrett and, 62, 66, 67, 72, 117; examines Elizabeth Garrett, 73; his lessons to Elizabeth Garrett, 76; leaves the Middlesex Hospital, *ib.*; alluded to, 80, 113; and the students' memorial against Elizabeth Garrett, 81; and the *Lancet* article, 85; a letter to Elizabeth Garrett quoted, *ib.*; discusses the examination at Apothecaries' Hall, 88; and St. Mary's Dispensary, 242
Pollock, Mr. A. G., 249, 250
Pollock, Sir Frederick, supports Elizabeth Garrett's candidature for School Board, 147
Portman Rooms (Baker Street), The, Elizabeth Garrett attends medical lectures at, 42
Powell, Dr., 111, 112, 113
Prince and Princess of Wales, The (after King Edward VII and Queen Alexandra), 236, 238, 247, 265
Princess Elizabeth of York Hospital for Children, The, alluded to, 128
Procter, Miss Adelaide Ann, 91; a biographical note of, *app.* 305, 306

Prostitutes, European methods with, 127
Punch, quoted, on the School Board election, *app.* 284

Qualifications for Women Act, The, 272
Queen's College for Women (Harley Street), The, 69; Sophia Jex-Blake at, 206

Railways, The, 23, 24
Ramsay, Miss Agnata, 232
Red Cross, The British, 275
Red Cross, The French, Mr. Norton a surgeon with, 138
Reform Bill, The, Elizabeth Garrett and, 38; of 1867, 121; Mill's amendment to, 122, 123
Richmond and Gordon, The Duke of, 221
'Riot of Surgeons' Hall' (Edinburgh), The, 208, 209
Robertson, Lady, 11, 250
Rome, Elizabeth Garrett Anderson goes to, 193; letters from, 194–6; alluded to, 203, 204
Rosa Morison Home of Recovery (Barnet), The, and Miss Morison, 250
Royal Free Hospital, The, refuses recognition of the London School of Medicine for Women, 219; the Chairman of the General Committee and the London School of Medicine, 223, 224; its alliance with the London School of Medicine for Women, 236; Miss Aldrich Blake and the museum of, 237; New Hospital for Women students and, 239

333

Index

Royal National Lifeboat Institution, The, 36
Rugby School, 32
Russell, Lord Provost Alexander, 209
Russell, The Countess, 10
Russell, Earl, 10, 160; a biographical note of, *app.* 306
Russia, 275

St. Andrews, University of, Elizabeth Garrett and matriculation at, 87, 89, *app.* 281, 282; alluded to, 90; medical examinations for women and, 97; Elizabeth Garrett goes to, *ib.*; her letters from, 98 *et seq.*; the matriculation ticket of, 99, 101; the Senatus of, 99, 101, 102, 103, 105; Elizabeth Garrett a member of, 100; Elizabeth Garrett and a likely lawsuit against, 103, 104
St. Bartholomew's Hospital, 244
St. George's Hall, Elizabeth Garrett's meeting in, 150, 153; London School of Medicine for Women appeal meeting at, 225
St. Leonard's, Louisa Garrett Anderson's school and mistress at, 266
St. Mary's College (St. Andrews), 103
St. Mary's Dispensary (after New Hospital for Women), started by Elizabeth Garrett, 120, 241; Elizabeth Garrett's work at, 241, 242 & *n.*, renamed New Hospital for Women, 242
St. Mary's Hospital, 241
St. Pancras, 150, 156, 246
Sanderson, Dr. Burdon, 216

Sandon, Lord, 159
Sant (artist), Mr., 161
Sargent, J. S., Elizabeth Garrett Anderson's portrait painted by, 270
Scharlieb, Mrs. Mary, and the London University, 232; the record of, 233; received by Queen Victoria and Prince and Princess of Wales, 236; goes to Madras, *ib.*; and the New Hospital for Women, 245; and drawing-room meetings for New Hospital for Women, 247
School Board, the London, Elizabeth Garrett and, 146, 147; Elizabeth Garrett's supporters for election to, 147, 148; Elizabeth Garrett's speeches as candidate for, 149 *et seq.*; Elizabeth Garrett's victory in election to, 154, 155, 185; the first meeting of, 156; Elizabeth Garrett and the chairmanship of, 158, 159; a painting of the first meeting of alluded to, 161; Elizabeth Garrett attends committees of, 179; Elizabeth Garrett Anderson retires from committee of, 191; *Punch*, on election for, *app.* 284
Schools, Elizabeth Garrett sent to Blackheath, 32; the Academy for Daughters of Gentlemen (Blackheath), 32, 33; Sunday, 40, elementary, 146
Scotland, the universities of, 96; Elizabeth Garrett in, 97 *et seq.*; Elizabeth Garrett's letters from, 98 *et seq.*; the Established Church Disruption (1843) in, 144; Rev. Alexander Anderson's house-

Index

hold in, 144, 145; Elizabeth Garrett on the auxiliary verbs 'shall' and 'will', in, 155, 156; Elizabeth Garrett's preference for the Church of, 168

Sedan, 139, 140, 141

Seely, Mrs., 195, 196

Sellar, Professor William Young, and wife of, 104 & n.

Seymour Place, the St. Mary's Dispensary in, 120, 241, 243

Shaftesbury, The Earl of, alluded to, 219, 222, 225; his humanitarian work alluded to, 219, 220; and the New Hospital for Women, 242; a biographical note of, (*Life* cited), *app.* 306, 307

Shelley, P. B., 203

Shove, Miss Edith., 222, 226, 232

Sidgwick, Henry, supports Elizabeth Garrett's candidature for School Board, 147, 148; a biographical note of, *app.* 307

Simpson (Edinburgh), Professor James Young, 107; a biographical note of, *app.* 307

Slader, Mr. Elizabeth Garrett's election expenses and, 160

Smith, Miss Annie Leigh, Emily Davies meets, 41; the education of, *ib.*; alluded to, 63; Elizabeth Garrett asks advice of, 71

Smith, Miss Barbara Leigh (*see* Bodichon, Mme)

Smith (advocate), Mr. Campbell, 105

Smith, Mr. James, 36, 63, 71, 72

Smith, Mrs. J.W., alluded to, 26, 32, 47, 67, 71, 85, 91, 115, 118, 206, 268; leaves the Academy at Blackheath, 33; at Alde House,

34; the marriage of, 36; visits school friends at Gateshead, 39, removes to Manchester Square; 72; Elizabeth Garrett at the house of, 73, 90, 107, 113; letters from Elizabeth Garrett to, 98–106; death of, 125; Elizabeth Garrett's love for, *ib.*; Elizabeth Garrett and the children of, 170, 179

Smith, Mrs. Sarah, 63

Smith, Sidney, 136

Smith, Sir Thomas, 241, 244, 249

Smith, Mr. Valentine, 42

Somerville, Mrs. Mary, 93; a biographical note of, *app.* 308

South Audley Street, Elizabeth Garrett removes to, 63; letters from, *ib.*

Spanish Armada, The, Aldeburgh and, 27

Spectator, The, 103, *app.* 281, 282

Spencer, Herbert, 124

Spurgeon, Charles Haddon, his *Sermons* alluded to, 29

Standard, The, 226

Stanley, Dean A. P., 158, a biographical note of (*Life* cited), *app.* 308

Stanley, Lady Augusta, *Letters* of, cited, *app.* 308

Stanley of Alderley, The Dowager Lady, 219; a biographical note of, *app.* 308, 309

Stansfeld, Rt. Hon. Sir James, and the Contagious Diseases Acts, 127; alluded to, 221, 225; his introduction to the London School of Medicine for Women, 223; meets Elizabeth Garrett Anderson, *ib.*; telegram to Miss

335

Index

Jex-Blake quoted, 224; a biographical note of (*Life* cited), *app.* 309, 310

Stephen, Lady, alluded to, 9, 91, 92, 121, 149; *Emily Davies and Girton College*, 9, 91, 92, *app.* 287, 289, 293

Sterilization, 53

Stevenson, Miss Flora, 146

Stevenson, Miss Louisa, 209

Stewart, Dr. A. P., 79, 257

Stewart-Wilson, Lady, 10

Strachey, Mrs. Oliver, 10

Strachey, Ray, *The Cause* cited, *app.* 295, *app.* 305

Struthers, Dr., 254

Sturgis, Dr., 216

Suffrage, Women's (*see* Women's Movement)

Surgery, the Middlesex Hospital ward of, 52; mortality of (1860), *ib.*; the conduct of, 53; and 'Listerism', *ib.*; Lister reforms procedure of, 54; Elizabeth Garrett Anderson at New Hospital for Women, 243, 244, 245; an ovariotomy operation by a woman, 244; Mrs. Scharlieb and, 245

Tate (schoolmaster), Mr., Elizabeth Garrett coached by, 44

Taylor, Miss Helen, 124, 135

Taylor, Mr., the chemistry lectures of, 76

Taylor, Mrs. Pet, 135

Temple, Rt. Hon. W. Cowper, 222

Tennyson, Lord, 138

The Times, 37, 160, 238; Elizabeth Garrett Anderson's letter on women students, 211, 212;

Sophia Jex-Blake replies to Elizabeth Garrett Anderson in, 212, 213

Thompson, Dr., Elizabeth Garrett and, 77; admits Elizabeth Garrett to his lectures, 78; and the Medical Schools' rejection of Elizabeth Garrett, 84

Thompson, Sir Henry and Lady, 143, 147

Thomson, Dr. H. Campbell, 10, 11

Thomson, Sir St. Clair, alluded to, 11; his tribute to Lister, 54; quoted, on Erichsen, 54, 55

Thomson & Co., George, 146

Thorne, Mrs. Isabel, alluded to, 210, 215, 222; appointed Hon. Sec. of London School of Medicine for Women, 227; Miss Jex-Blake's letter to, resigning trusteeship, 228

Thorold, Mr., 155, 159

Todd, Dr. Margaret, *Life of Sophia Jex-Blake*, cited, 210; quoted, 212, 215, 223, 224, 228, *app.* 300, 301, 309, 310

Trelawney, Edward John, 203; a biographical note of, *app.* 310

Tulloch (St. Andrews), Dr., his support of Elizabeth Garrett, 101, 102

Turle, Mr., 239, 249

Ufford (Suffolk), 25; a letter of Elizabeth Garrett's quoted, 45

United Colleges of St. Salvator and St. Leonard (St. Andrews), The, 103

University College Medical School, 55

336

Index

Upper Berkeley Street, No. 20, leased for Elizabeth Garrett, 118; the franchise meetings at, 121; alluded to, 170, 171; letters from, 170, 174, 178, 179

Vallory-Radot, R., *Life of Pasteur* quoted, 53, 54
Venice, 205
Vere Street Chapel, Elizabeth Garrett attends, 68, 110
Victoria, Princess, 247
Victoria, Queen, Elizabeth Garrett's early recollection of, 26; alluded to, 130, 191; Miss Beilby and, 235; and *purdah*, ib., opposes women in medicine, ib.; receives Mrs. Scharlieb, 236; her death alluded to, 265; Henry Fawcett's *faux pas* towards, 265
Votes for Women movement, The, beginning of (1867), 18; alluded to, 273, 274; Elizabeth Garrett Anderson and, 274

Wade, Dr., 257
Walker, Dr., 139, 248
Wandsworth, 182
War of 1914, The, Elizabeth Garrett Anderson and, 275; the first medical unit for, ib.
Waterston, Miss Jane, 218
Wedgewood, Miss Julia, supports Elizabeth Garrett's candidature for School Board, 147
Wells (artist), Mr., 161
Wells, Sir Spencer, 245
West Brompton, Elizabeth Garrett Anderson at hospital of, 198
Westlake, Mrs., 148

Westminster, the parliamentary candidate for (1865), 120; alluded to, 160
Whitby, 223
Whitehills (Aberdeenshire), 145
Willis, Dr., discusses training with Elizabeth Garrett, 59; Elizabeth Garrett's appreciation of kindness of, 62; advises a tutor for Elizabeth Garrett, 70, 72; his first lesson to Elizabeth Garrett, 72; examines Elizabeth Garrett, 73; alluded to, 77
Wimbledon, Mr. Anderson in camp at, 142; Elizabeth Garrett visits the camp at, ib.
Wimpole Street, No. 69, offices of the London School of Medicine for Women at, 216
Windsor Castle, 33, 236
Wollstonecraft, Mary, *A Vindication of the Rights of Women* alluded to, 17; the work for women of, 17, 18; death of, 18
Women, position in England of, 17-24; Mary Wollstonecraft and, 17, 18; and the Humanitarian movement, 18; beginning of organized movement for, ib.; demand for votes for, ib.; the marriage disabilities of (1836), 19; unmarried, ib.; education of, 20; sports and dress of, 20, 21; the repression of, (1836), 21, 22; the intellectual status of, 22; Elizabeth Garrett's protests for, 23; the bicycle and dress reform for, 24; Emily Davies and the position of, 40, 41; physicians, 51; and speeches, 149; the London School of

Index

Medicine for (*vide*); American physicians, 207; and the Hope Scholarship award, 208; Faculty of Medicine (Edin.), hostility to, 208; and the Medical Register, 210; and the British Medical Association, 251 *et seq.*; and Votes for, 273, 274; and the War of 1914, 275; and matriculation, *app.* 282

Women's Enfranchisement Petition (1866), The, Elizabeth Garrett and, 122

Women's Hospital Corps, The, in the War of 1914, 275

Women's Movement, The, the beginning of, 17, 18; *A Vindication of the Rights of Women* alluded to, *ib.*; Mary Wollstonecraft and, 17, 18; and Elizabeth Garrett, 18; legal disabilities of married women (1836), and, 19; early support gained for, 23; Emily Davies and, 39, 40; Mr. and Mrs. Russell Gurney and, 84; Elizabeth Garrett's enthusiasm in, 90, 91; Miss Jane Crowe and, 91; Mme Bodichon's bureau, 91; the enfranchisement,

121-4; the first debate on the suffrage, 123; Elizabeth Garrett's part in, 134; supporters of, 147, 148; the School Board election victory and, 155, 161; and Elizabeth Garrett's engagement, 164; Sophia Jex-Blake and, 207, 208; and the Edinburgh University hostility to, 209; and Votes for Women, 273; parliamentary support of, 274; Mrs. and Miss Pankhurst and, *ib.*

Wordsworth, William, the poems of, 142

Working Class, the, Elizabeth Garrett addresses, 151; and the School Board election, 156

Working Men's Association, The, 147

Working Men's College, The, the Rifle Corps, 74, 75

Worthington, Dr., 60

Yarrow (matron), Mrs., 59
York, 197

Zürich, the M.D. degree of, 210, 242, 243, 256

www.ingramcontent.com/pod-product-compliance
Ingram Content Group UK Ltd.
Pitfield, Milton Keynes, MK11 3LW, UK
UKHW040658180125
453697UK00010B/258

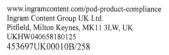

9 781108 079280